How To
Help Him

How To
Help Him

The Book for Women
Worried About a Man

Ryan Parke

First published in 2025 by Intellectual Perspective Press

© Copyright Ryan Parke

All rights reserved. No part of this publication may be reproduced, stored in or introduced into a retrieval system, or transmitted, in any form, or by any means (electronic, mechanical, photocopying, recording or otherwise) without the prior written permission of the Publisher.

The right of Ryan Parke to be identified as the author of this work has been asserted in accordance with the Copyright, Designs and Patents Act 1988.

This book is sold subject to the condition that it shall not, by way of trade or otherwise, be lent, resold, hired out, or otherwise circulated without the publisher's prior consent in any form of binding or cover other than that in which it is published and without a similar condition including this condition being imposed on the subsequent Purchaser.

The purpose of this book is to educate and entertain. The author and Intellectual Perspective Press shall have neither liability nor responsibility to any person or entity with respect to any loss or damage caused, or alleged to have been caused, directly or indirectly, by the information contained in this book.

Book Interior and E-book Design by Amit Dey (amitdey2528@gmail.com)

To find out more about our authors and books visit: www.intellectualperspective.com

TABLE OF CONTENTS

Content notice xiii
Praise for How to Help Him xv
PART 1: The Current Approach to Mental Health is not Working for Men 1
    Brad's story 1
    The day heart attacks jump up in men 4
    The 5 Dimensions of male mental health 14
    How to use this book 20
PART 2: Achieving Recognition 27
    Achieving Recognition: Signs of stress 27
        –Feeling "stuck" or unsuccessful 27
        –Lack of written goals 27
        –Outcome-based goals 27
        –Comparison with others 27
        –Loss of social status (redundancy, retirement) 27
    Christopher's story 27
    Achieving Recognition: The science 31
        The risk is not spread evenly amongst men 31
        Serotonin: The "good news" neurotransmitter 35
        Serotonin: How males track social status 36
        Sense of success: The 2 factors that make it 39
        The way we set goals often makes things worse 41

Achieving Recognition: Strategies 43
    ❑ Write down life goals 43
    ❑ Identify obstacles 44
    ❑ Set weekly goals 44
    ❑ Weekly goals should be small, effort-based, and wholly within your control... 45
    ❑ Arrange weekly accountability 45

PART 3: Looking After Body & Mind 49
Looking After Body & Mind: Signs of stress 49
    -Feeling down, depressed 49
    -Low energy, poor sleep 49
    -Poor prostate health 49
    -High blood pressure 49
    -Poor heart health 49
    -Type 2 diabetes 49
    -Low libido, ED 49
Steve's story 49
Looking After Body & Mind: The science 54
    The decline of testosterone 54
    Why low testosterone is so dangerous for men................ 56
    How low-carb impacts testosterone in men 59
    How low-fat and low cholesterol impact life expectancy 65
    Testosterone: The male "capability" hormone 74
Looking After Body & Mind: Strategies............................... 79
    ❑ Real food: reduce carbohydrates; increase natural fats 79
    ❑ Sleep: 7-8 hours per day 81
    ❑ Exercise: 150 minutes / week..................................... 82
    ❑ Vitamin D3: sunlight, supplements, natural fat 84

- ❏ Reduce / stop drinking alcohol 85
- ❏ Watch team wins 86

PART 4: Protecting the Cave 95

Protecting the Cave: Signs of stress 95
- -Feeling overwhelmed 95
- -Feeling hopeless or ashamed 95
- -Financial uncertainty... 95
- -Relationship insecurity... 95
- -Feeling like a burden 95

Gary's story... 95

Protecting the Cave: The science 100
- Financial security and male mental health........................ 100
- How improving financial security impacts male mental health 102
- Relationship security and male mental health 105
- Oxytocin: The hormone that bonds us............................ 107
- Oxytocin: The hormone that divides us........................... 110

Protecting the Cave: Strategies 116
- ❏ Express and address underlying issues 116
- ❏ Review monthly costs 116
- ❏ Focus on building a monthly surplus............................ 117
- ❏ Team up with money / debt charities (if needed)................ 118
- ❏ Spend quality time with partner (if relevant) 118

PART 5: Having Adventures... 121

Having Adventures: Signs of stress 121
- -Life flying by... 121
- -Lack of motivation 121
- -Working all the time.. 121
- -Procrastination 121

- Distractions / cravings (eg: porn, alcohol, social media, etc.) 121

Ryan's story 121

Having Adventures: The science 127

    Dopamine: The molecule of motivation 127

    Dopamine: The chemical of craving 131

    Things that "spike" dopamine 132

    How dopamine dysregulation impacts motivation
        and discipline 140

    Restoring motivation and discipline 144

Having Adventures: Strategies 150

    ❏ Take time to 'recharge' 150

    ❏ Explore new places and skills 151

    ❏ Identify distractions 151

    ❏ Cut out / get help with distractions 152

    ❏ Use smartphone in black and white mode 152

PART 6: Able to Serve 157

Able to Serve: Signs of stress 157

    - Feeling useless 157

    - Feeling unfulfilled 157

    - Wondering what is the point of life? 157

    - Loss of child contact 157

    - Death feels meaningful or heroic 157

Jaden's story 157

Able to Serve: The science 162

    It's not a lack of talking or talking therapy 162

    Why the current approach might not be enough
        to tackle male suicide 165

    Men are talking; but are we listening? 171

    How masculinity impacts male mental health 175

When life lacks purpose, death feels meaningful 184

Able to Serve: Strategies 187

❏ Identify skills and strengths 188

❏ Serve people / causes that matter most 189

❏ Support family, friends, and faith 189

❏ Be part of a team 191

❏ Say "no" to unfulfilling things 192

PART 7: It's about balance 197

PART 8: How to Talk to Him 199

Supporting connection 199

Supporting capability 201

During a personal crisis 202

Dealing with disappointment 206

Talking about dangerous driving 208

Encouraging boys (and men) to help with tasks 209

When to support connection and when to support
  capability 210

More supportive statements and questions 211

Recommended word swaps 213

How to help him to find the right support 216

Final thoughts 218

Next steps 220

Thank you page 210

How to test Testosterone Levels 221

1. How to test 221

2. When to test 221

3. Which markers to test 221

4. How often to test 222

    5. Which test to buy 222

    6. The problem with just testing 222

About Ryan Parke 223

The ALPHA Framework: Quick Reference Guide 224

Mental Health Support 225

Ryan's Resources page 226

CONTENT NOTICE

This book makes references to suicide. Suicide is preventable and support is available. What helps one person might not work for another, so don't give up. Some of the resources Ryan signposts to are listed at TheMensCoach.co.uk/resources – or scan the QR code below and tap 'Resources'.

This book focuses on male mental health; however, everyone's mental health is important and anyone can have thoughts of suicide regardless of their biological sex or gender identity.

Ryan wrote this book for women because the vast majority of people who have asked him for a book are women worried about a man in their life. However, if you're not a woman — perhaps a dad, son, brother, friend, non-binary person, or man in a same-sex relationship — you are very welcome here, and Ryan believes much of what he shares will still be useful to you.

Gender identity is distinct from biological sex. Everyone's experiences and identities are valid and respected as we explore this topic together. Throughout this book, the terms "*men*" and "*males*" may be used interchangeably, depending on the context. This is to stay consistent with the language used in the research, which often uses the term "*men*" to refer to people who were assigned male at birth. Unless indicated otherwise, the science discussed in this book applies to people with a typical male hormonal profile, which may include trans women and non-binary people who were assigned male at birth (AMAB).

The aim of this book is to make relevant scientific discoveries available to everyone, along with strategies that have worked for men on Ryan's coaching programme. None of the information in this book is intended to replace personalised advice you may have received based on your individual circumstances.

This is the UK edition of this book, but content may vary by region. Please consider whether you are comfortable reading a UK edition before proceeding, as cultural values and sensitivities may differ around the world.

If you have a medical condition, mental health condition, or take medication, speak to your healthcare provider before using the information in this book.

PRAISE FOR HOW TO HELP HIM

If you want to understand and help your male partner, friend, child, or family member this is the book for you! Ryan Parke has put his heart and soul into this book to bring to us the wisdom of his knowledge and research. 'How to Help Him' is very thought provoking and some information could be a light bulb moment for many readers. A book I would definitely recommend.

— Jenny Rayner, CEO,
The Lucy Rayner Foundation

A compassionate and practical guide for anyone worried about a man in their life. Evidence-based and deeply human. I've used some of these approaches in my own therapy practice and have seen firsthand how effective they are. This book doesn't just explain how to help — it gives readers the tools and confidence to make a real difference.

— Jamie Compton-Rea MBACP,
Integrative Therapist and Chief Operations Officer
at National Centre for Suicide Prevention Education & Training CIC

You will find things in this book to inspire you, to challenge you, and to help you better understand, support and empower the people you care about.

— Dr Fiona Rogers, Deputy CEO,
Council of British International Schools (COBIS)

A perfect resource for educators, therapists, professionals parents but most importantly anyone in today's society - that is Ryan's biggest strength; making such vital information accessible to all!

— George Peterkin, Educator,
Eating disorder therapist, and founder of Mind Your Health Ltd.

Thanks to Ryan's work, I can truly see, hear, and support the men in my life in ways I never could before. How to Help him is a game changer.

– *Zoie Golding MBE,*
Founder of The Big Movement by ZoieLogic

Arm yourself with the knowledge and tools in this book. You'll not only strengthen the bond with your man, but also witness the transformation as he finds his way back to his best self.

– *Nick Burnett, Co-Founder & CEO, Selph*

Ryan's approach is a game-changer for anyone who has concerns about the mental health of the men they care about.

– *Shirley Heapy, Trustee, The Clive Smith Foundation;*
ESG Manager, Baily Garner LLP

A groundbreaking, evidence-based roadmap, to help you support the men and boys in your life, Ryan has created a first class resource which will no doubt improve the wellbeing of many men and ultimately save lives. It's packed with practical strategies and is easy to read, written in a down-to-earth, accessible style.

– *Andrew Pain, TEDx & CPD Accredited Speaker on*
Men's Mental Health, Burnout and Work-Life Balance

As a woman who cares deeply about all the great men in my life, I found this book to be a real game-changer. I feel like I now know how to be there in a way that makes a true difference. And you can't put a price on that.

– *Dani Wallace,*
Founder of The BIG Festoon and CEO of IATQB

Genuinely superb. If you have a man in your life who you care about, this book should be your next purchase.

– *Mark Leppard MBE,*
Headmaster at The British School Al Khubairat,
Abu Dhabi; Chairman of British Schools in
the Middle East (BSME); SchoolsCompare.com's
Best Principal in the UAE 2023

A guide to finding your own strength, and balance in supporting them as a compassionate companion.

> – *Ann Millington OBE QFSM,*
> *CEO of Kent Fire and Rescue Service*

Reading this book feels like someone is taking your hand and saying, 'You're not alone, and there are things you can do that really matter.' If you're worried about a man in your life and don't know how to reach him, this book is the lifeline you've been searching for. I truly believe this book will change and even save lives!

> – *Lauren Rimmer,*
> *Founder & CEO, Construct Change*

PART 1:

THE CURRENT APPROACH TO MENTAL HEALTH IS NOT WORKING FOR MEN

Brad's story

In June 2019, I bumped into a lady I hadn't seen in years, and I was really excited to hear the latest about her son.

Jenny's son, Brad, was taller than me, more muscular, and slightly better looking. Brad had a fast car, a big house, and a great job. Plus, he was a dad with a loving wife.

And at the time, I liked to think that I was on the same trajectory as Brad – just a couple of years behind because of the age difference.

Then I saw the look on his mum's face, and I wondered what I had said to upset her. "*How's Brad?*" Jenny repeated. "*Ryan, you don't know…? Brad's taken his own life.*"

She closed her eyes, and a tear rolled down her cheek. We stood in silence for a moment under the hornbeam trees outside Jenny's house, on a summer afternoon.

At the time, it didn't make sense to me.

I was really taken aback by this news for 2 main reasons. First was the loss of Brad. I couldn't believe that he was gone. At the time I had preconceived ideas that things like this didn't happen to men like Brad.

But there was another reason, too, that Brad's death was deeply concerning to me. Until that day, I had always heard and believed that the reason why men have higher rates of suicide than women is because *men don't talk*, and *they don't reach out for help*.

And yet Brad was the most open and articulate man I knew...

Jenny broke the silence and shakily shared with me that, years before Brad's death, he had decided to reach out for help with his mental health. One of the ways that Brad did this was to visit his doctor.

Brad's doctor did what doctors are trained to do and referred him to talking therapy and prescribed antidepressants.

Brad attended different forms of talking therapy, and took antidepressants. Two months before his death, Jenny – who works in mental health herself – said, "Brad, call me every night, tell me how you feel. You've got to get these feelings off your chest."

Now, don't get me wrong. I'm not suggesting these things didn't help Brad. I am sure that they did. But what struck me at the time was that here was a man who had done all the things that we tell men in crisis to do (seek help, talk about how you feel), and yet he still didn't survive. I wondered what else Brad could have done?

Standing under the trees outside her house, Jenny told me the following fact:

Every 5 hours, 4 people die from suicide in the UK and Ireland. Three of them are going to be men. To put that into perspective, that's roughly a double-decker bus full of men every 4 days in the UK and Ireland alone. The age group often most at risk is men aged from their mid-30s to their late 40s. [1][2][3]

Since records began in 1861, Jenny told me, more men have died from suicide every year in the UK than women. [4]

I asked Jenny what I could do to help. She told me to set some time aside to learn about male mental health. And if I wanted to make a difference, to donate some money to a local suicide prevention charity (The OLLIE Foundation) who she had found extremely helpful.[5]

As I walked home, I couldn't forget the look of pain in Jenny's eyes, and the silence that had filled the air. I knew I had to do something, but I didn't know what. I was not a mental health practitioner. At the time, I actually believed that "mental health" didn't affect me. After this encounter, I was starting to realise that I was wrong, and decided to start by setting aside some time to learn about the subject. Sunday afternoons would now be dedicated to male mental health research. If nothing else, I could educate myself to hopefully reduce the chance that one day it would be my mum standing under the hornbeam trees, saying that she had lost her son.

If you're reading this book then, like Jenny, you are worried about a man in your life. Like Jenny, you're probably prepared to do anything you can to help. But unlike Jenny, I don't ever want you to feel the pain of losing him.

Jenny knew something was wrong. She felt it in her gut. She knew Brad was in trouble. At first, she felt the frustration of seeing Brad not reach out for help when she felt he needed it.

But then she experienced a new horror. Jenny saw Brad reaching out time and time again for help, which just didn't work for him. In the years, months, and weeks leading up to his death, Jenny began to live a waking nightmare. She could see first-hand that the support available just wasn't working for Brad. She had seen this happen to other men in her own career in mental health; seeing her son on the same path was the hardest experience of her life.

Brad's death and Jenny's experience are both tragedies, but they are not isolated incidents. Jenny's harrowing fact tells us that around the world, the vast majority of those who take their own lives are male. This is often attributed to men *"not reaching out for help"*, but over the course of this book, I want to show you that this oversimplification is distracting from the real challenges that men face. I want to show you that there are practical solutions to the challenges that men face, but you don't find them unless you really dig deep and know what to look for.

Whether you are a mum, wife, partner, sister, friend, or colleague worried about a man in your life, this book is for you. I want to take what I learned on my journey and repurpose it so that, rather than offering practical strategies to just men, I can offer practical steps to the women who support them, and an explanation as to why the steps work.

As you'll have gathered by now, I make multiple references to suicide. If this is a sensitive topic for you, this might not be the right book for you at the moment. But I believe it's important for us to understand the factors associated with male suicide – because once we do, we can see why a one-size-fits-all approach to mental health isn't working for men, and what needs to change.

Having had conversations with women who are concerned about the men in their lives, suicide is often at the forefront of their minds due to its increasing coverage in the media. But even if (and I hope this is the case), he is not having thoughts about suicide, the strategies in this book will allow you to understand and support him better than before.

It's possible that some of the steps in this book might not be relevant or appropriate to your situation. But that doesn't mean the knowledge isn't worth having for the future. I've tried to lay out the book so that you can go to the bits that feel most relevant, and take what you need.

I've been where you might be now – feeling like you don't know how to help. Jenny helped me to get started by telling me to do some research. So I did. A lot of research. I'll share those first few weeks of research with you now, so you can see where my approach and theories all started. This starting point is often a surprise to most people who hear it, but I promise it will all come together and make sense.

The day heart attacks jump up in men

The following Sunday was my first day dedicated to researching male mental health. I didn't really know where to start, so I decided to first understand more about life expectancy in men. I thought that by understanding more about the biggest killers of men, I would get an understanding of where to start when it came to the impact of mental health on men's lives.

I quickly learned that the biggest killers of UK men vary by age: [6]

- Until age 50: suicide
- Age 50–79: heart disease, followed by cancer
- Over age 80: Alzheimer's disease and dementia

I decided that – in order to take a holistic approach – I should keep my eyes, ears, and mind open to information on heart disease, cancer, and Alzheimer's, those top 3 killers of men over the age of 50. I began to search for relevant studies on life expectancy in men, using websites like PubMed and Google Scholar to read articles that had been published in peer reviewed scientific journals.

About 4 hours into my search, I read something that really jumped out at me:

Every year, there's a day when heart attacks in men increase by as much as 30%, while on the same day, heart attacks in women appear to decrease slightly. [7][8][9]

The day in question is the Monday after the clocks jump forwards by 1 hour (known as the beginning of "daylight savings time"). In the UK and US, this is in March each year. In Australia, this is in October.

And when I first learned this, I was compelled to find out more. After all, how could the same thing (a change in the clocks) impact men and women in such radically different ways? I spent the rest of that day reading around this phenomenon, to see whether I could understand why these clock changes cause such different effects in men versus women.

Unfortunately, I couldn't find any studies or articles that could answer my question directly. But I did learn some new things that I thought seemed very relevant.

When the clocks jump forwards, we should really all go to bed an hour early to avoid missing sleep. But have you ever actually done that? No, me neither. And neither do most people. This means that in countries where there is a clock change, it's like a mass science experiment each year where almost everyone in the country loses an hour of sleep at the same time.

What happens in your body when you lose even one hour's sleep depends upon whether you're biologically male or biologically female. For men, several studies have suggested that lost sleep can negatively impact their testosterone levels, and other studies have found that – in a male body – as testosterone goes down, the chances of having a heart attack go up. [10] [11] [12] [13]

When I first learned about a potential link between *low testosterone* and *heart attacks* in men, I was quite surprised. Because at that point in my life, I had never heard anything positive about testosterone. In fact, I remember when I was a child and there was a fight in the playground or my local pub, my parents' friends used to say "*It's no wonder they ended up fighting. There was **too much testosterone**.*" Testosterone, I had always thought, was a hormone that makes men and boys aggressive.

So I wondered: how can a hormone known for causing fights also protect a man's heart against a heart attack? By the time I reached that thought, however, I had been reading studies non-stop for hours and I was tired. But next Sunday, I would have to learn more about this hormone, testosterone.

As the following Sunday came around, it was time for my second day of research. And my first research question was: "*Why does testosterone make men aggressive?*"

I quickly learned that testosterone does *not* make men aggressive. Studies that have investigated this stereotype have found there is no reason to believe that natural levels of testosterone makes men aggressive (however high). [14] [15] [16]

Despite testosterone's notoriety as an "angry hormone", there are lots of reasons to believe the opposite is true. Studies on men and other animals have found that testosterone has a calming effect on males. [17] [18] [19]

As it turns out, the early studies that gave testosterone its bad reputation weren't even based on natural testosterone levels. They were based on observing what happened when men inject very high levels of testosterone, which isn't the same thing. Based on what I learned, I realised that we can safely let go of the assumption that *testosterone makes men aggressive.* [20]

Now, knowing that testosterone doesn't cause aggression, my next question was: *"Why does testosterone seem to protect a man from having a heart attack?"* [21]

But while trying to investigate the links between testosterone and heart health in men, I kept finding links to studies on male mental health. Firstly, how poor heart health in men seems to coincide with depression. Secondly, how both poor heart health and depression seem to coincide with having low testosterone.

Multiple studies have found that low testosterone in men is associated with, and predicts, depression. One study of middle-aged depressed men found that their testosterone levels are 32% lower than men who are not depressed. [22] [23] [24] [25] And many high quality clinical trials have found that increasing testosterone significantly reduces depression symptoms in men. [26]

This made me really want to drill down into testosterone in much greater detail. What is a "healthy" level of testosterone? How low is "low"? And how had I got to age 29 without hearing about this before?

Let's look at what I found, one thing at a time.

Firstly, what is a "healthy level"?

Testosterone in the blood is very easy to measure. A 2017 analysis published in *The Journal of Clinical Endocrinology & Metabolism* took data from 4 famous studies and found that the (median) average level of testosterone for healthy, non-obese men aged 18 to 39 is **18.4 nmol/L**. [27]

So let's use 18.4 nmol/L as our "healthy" standard for testosterone levels in men.

Compare this with testosterone levels in depressed middle-aged men, which tend to be more like 11.9 nmol/L. That's quite a big difference. This made me start to wonder whether there was a relationship between low testosterone and suicide. [28]

In 2007, researchers compared the testosterone levels of men with mental health conditions who had previous attempted suicide with the testosterone levels of those without mental health conditions or thoughts about suicide. They found that men who had recently attempted suicide had much lower levels of testosterone than men who did not have thoughts about suicide. They also found that – when you compared testosterone levels of the men who had attempted suicide – lower levels of testosterone were associated with more violent methods, and with more past suicide attempts. In the men who had attempted suicide in the most violent ways, the average level of testosterone was just 8.8 nmol/L – 52% *lower than the healthy average of 18.4 nmol/L.* [29]

A year later, the same researchers repeated their findings, this time comparing men who had needed hospital care after surviving a suicide attempt, with those who had needed hospital care after an accidental injury. Again, the men who had attempted suicide had lower levels of testosterone. [30]

Then, in 2021, a small study on male military veterans used a questionnaire to calculate SSI scores (a way of measuring how strongly someone is thinking about suicide) and then compared the results to their testosterone levels. The study found that lower testosterone levels were associated with higher SSI scores across the whole group. The lower the testosterone in these men, the more strongly the association with suicide. [31]

And a much older study, published in *Psychological Reports* in 1986, measured the testosterone levels in the bodies of men who had sadly taken their own lives. This study found that average levels of testosterone found in the men who had died from suicide was just 11.7 nmol/L. The average age of these men was only 39. As you'll see in part 3 of this book, 11.7 nmol/L was extremely low back in 1986 – much lower than it seems now, as testosterone levels in men were generally much higher then. [32]

Unfortunately, the team who carried out this study didn't seem to realise what they had found. Rather than comparing 11.7 nmol/L to healthy men, they compared the testosterone levels of the male suicide victims with men who died from a sudden death (like a pulmonary disorder). And the sudden death group had even lower levels of testosterone at 8.4 nmol/L. This led the authors of this study to state that men who died from suicide had "higher" levels of testosterone.

In the decades since, this 1986 study seems to have led to a belief that *"higher testosterone levels are associated with suicide in younger men"*. But that's not what the 1986 study actually found, it's just that other articles seemed to take its comments at face value, without actually looking at the testosterone measurements from the study. [33][34][35]

It appears that both male suicide survivors and male suicide victims may have much *lower* levels of testosterone than healthy men. These studies on testosterone and suicide stunned me. Of all the articles and public health campaigns I had seen around suicide in men by this point, I'd never seen or heard anything to do with testosterone levels. But the fact that suicide is the biggest killer of men under 50, and men who think about, attempt, and even die from suicide seem to have low testosterone, it all seemed relevant.

But I didn't want to just stay there with the research. As relevant as the links were between low testosterone, depression and suicide in men were, I wanted to understand the wider picture. As we know, around the age of 50, the biggest killer of men moves from suicide to heart disease.

"Heart disease" isn't a specific illness. It's a collective term for many heart problems, including coronary artery disease, heart attack, heart failure, and others. And in men, coronary artery disease, heart attack, heart failure, and high blood pressure are all associated with having a low level of testosterone. [36][37]

In 1987, a study published in *Journal of the American Geriatrics Society* found that testosterone levels of 15.1 nmol/L and below were associated with heart attack in men aged 46 to 89. What's more, age had nothing to do with testosterone levels, but a history of heart problems or heavy drinking did. [38]

Later in this book, you'll see that even momentary dips in testosterone are associated with significant spikes in heart attack risk.

As Dr Travis Goodale et al. wrote in a 2017 article:

"Low testosterone levels in men may increase their risk of developing [heart disease], metabolic syndrome, and type 2 diabetes. Reduced testosterone levels

in men with congestive heart failure (CHF) [predict a worse outcome] and are associated with [a higher risk of death]." [39]

So, we can surmise that low testosterone appears to be a significant problem for a man's heart. But the association between low testosterone and shorter life expectancy doesn't end there.

After heart disease, the next biggest killer of men over the age of 50 is cancer. The most likely cancer that a UK or US man will be diagnosed with, by a long way, is prostate cancer – a cancer which disproportionately affects Black men more than other races. [40] [41] [42]

In a 2016 study published in *BJU International*, 681 men who underwent a prostate biopsy were divided into 2 groups: those with testosterone below 10.4 nmol/L ("low testosterone") and those with higher testosterone. Men with low testosterone had more than 2.5× the odds of being diagnosed with prostate cancer, and over 3.3× the odds of being diagnosed with an aggressive form of the disease. Even after adjusting for factors like age, prostate specific antigen (PSA) level, BMI, and diabetes, men with low testosterone still had over twice the odds of aggressive prostate cancer. [43] Another study showed that the longer a man can maintain a testosterone level of over 12.1 nmol/L, the lower his lifetime risk of developing prostate cancer. [44] [45]

Prostate cancer awareness campaigns are often focussed around PSA testing and I had always been told that the way to detect prostate cancer is having a blood test to check your PSA level. But there is evidence that focussing on PSA and ignoring testosterone is costing lives.

In 1996, 77 men who had been given the "all clear" after a PSA screening test and a manual prostate exam were called back to be re-examined because they had low testosterone. Eleven of the men (14%) were found to have prostate cancer that had not been detected by the PSA test or manual exam. In men over the age of 60, 30% had prostate cancer that had been missed by the PSA and prostate exam. The study concluded:

"These data suggest that digital rectal examination and PSA levels are insensitive indicators of prostate cancer in men with low total or free testosterone levels." [46]

That's not to say that PSA testing isn't a useful tool in detecting prostate cancer. It just suggests that PSA levels are more useful in those with a healthy level of testosterone.

And if a man does develop prostate cancer, his testosterone levels may also predict the outcome. In a study of men with advanced (stage 4) prostate cancer, testosterone was found to be a more accurate predictor of life expectancy than PSA levels, number of cancer sites, and concurrent diseases. The higher their testosterone levels, the longer they survived. The study also found that age plays a significant role: men diagnosed at an older age tended to survive longer after diagnosis than younger men. [47]

By the age of 80, the single biggest killer of men becomes Alzheimer's disease and dementia. And in older men, having a low level of active testosterone (often called "*free testosterone*") appears to precede the onset of Alzheimer's disease by about 6 years. Another study recommended that low testosterone in elderly men should be seen as a biomarker for "*cognitive decline and dementia, including Alzheimer's disease*". [48,49,50]

And multiple long-term studies have found that men with higher testosterone levels live longer; such studies include the National Health and Nutrition Examination Survey (NHANES) (10,225 Americans) and The Rancho Bernardo Study (6,000 Americans followed for 40+ years). [51,52]

Let's summarise what we've learned about testosterone so far:

- Until age 50, suicide is the biggest killer of UK men.
- In men, both suicide and depression in men are linked to low testosterone.
- Between ages 50 and 79, heart disease is the biggest killer of UK men.
- Heart disease is also the single biggest killer of men overall.
- In men, heart disease, heart attack, heart failure, and high blood pressure are all linked to having low testosterone.
- The next biggest killer of men over the age of 50 worldwide is cancer.

- The most common form of cancer in UK and US men (prostate cancer) is linked to low testosterone.
- After age 80, Alzheimer's and dementia are the biggest killers of UK men.
- In men, Alzheimer's disease and dementia are associated with low testosterone levels.
- Long-term studies show that men with higher testosterone levels live longer.

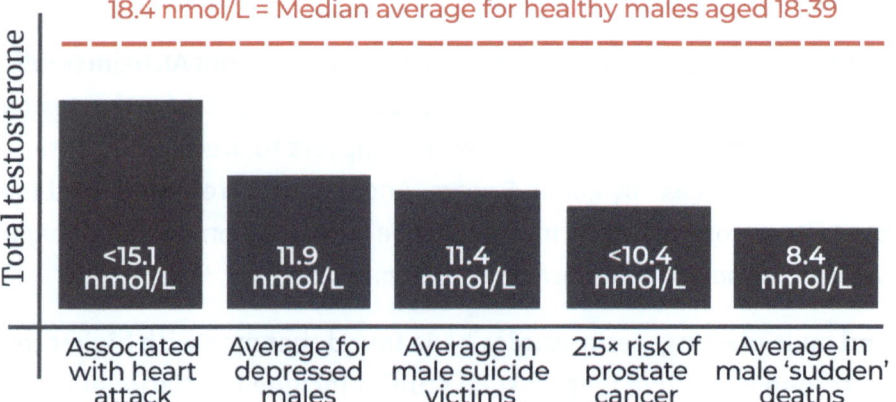

Adapted from: R556: T.G Travison et al. (2017); R561: C Swartz et al. (1987); R133: R McIntyre et al. (2006); R842: B Roland et al. (1986); R117: J Parke et al. (2016). Compiled by Ryan Parke. Full references in preceding text.

Now — before anyone says it — I am very aware that the relationship so far between low testosterone and the biggest killers of men is **correlation** (2 things happening at the same time) and not **causation** (one thing causing the other). And I **am not** suggesting that all men need to do is boost their testosterone levels and all their health issues will be solved. But during part 3 of this book, I will share a reason why men with low testosterone levels die sooner, and what to do about it.

The reason I have shared these studies so far is to show:

All the biggest killers of UK men today are associated with having a low level of testosterone. And yet men aren't told this.

What I didn't know at the time was:

1. Testosterone levels are constantly declining in developed countries.
2. Most men can easily improve testosterone levels through lifestyle alone.
3. Many GPs and mental health professionals receive little to no training on testosterone, and are often unaware of the research we've just explored.

After weeks of regular research, I had deduced that:

- testosterone was important for men;
- a healthy level of testosterone is around 18 nmol/L to 32 nmol/L;
- things tend to start going wrong for men once testosterone levels get below 16 nmol/L.

But when I looked at the "normal" reference ranges for testosterone, I was stunned.

In the UK, most labs that offer testosterone tests for men refer to testosterone levels of just 12 nmol/L and above as being "normal". The NHS app tends to draw the line at 11.7 nmol/L. And – at the point of publishing – several UK labs suggest that even 8.6 nmol/L is "optimal" for men under 50 (or 6.7 nmol/L in men over 50). [53]

This means that the men we care about could have a level of testosterone that is associated with depression, heart disease, prostate cancer, and Alzheimer's, and yet be told by a lab they trust that they have "optimal" levels of testosterone. To me, this seems dangerously misleading.

In the years since I first discovered the correlations between testosterone levels and men's health, many hormone experts have explained to me that the reference ranges used by labs have decreased in line with decreasing levels of testosterone in men in developed countries. It appears that healthcare providers and labs may be confusing "optimal" with normal. Given that we live in a world where it is 'normal' to develop depression, heart disease, and prostate cancer, it seems important to me that we can tell normal and optimal apart!

This is not a book purely about testosterone (although in part 3 I will explain why low testosterone is such a problem for men, and how men can quickly, naturally, and significantly improve testosterone levels). The reason I shared all this with you is because I wanted to immerse you in my experience of what I learned in my first few weeks of trying to learn about male mental health. I started out with beliefs I had never questioned – beliefs like *"testosterone makes men aggressive"* and *"men just need to talk"*. But the research painted an entirely different picture, and I could quickly see that stereotypes like this aren't only wrong; they might be dangerously misleading.

Not only is testosterone a vital health marker in men, but there is clearly more to male mental health than just talking. No amount of talking alone can fix a biological issue like low testosterone.

The 5 Dimensions of male mental health

You might find it strange that I dived so deep into research about testosterone. I suppose it was, though I was only doing what I had been taught to do in my work.

When I heard about Brad, I was the sales and operations director for a car finance brokerage I had co-founded when I was 23. With the help of an older, silent business partner, I had built a company with a great team, a good reputation, and reliable quarterly profits for 5 years.

Everything in our industry was quarterly. Every 3 months, every finance company would stop all of their offers, review their balance sheet, and start again. For brokers like us, there was a wild race to publicise the new offers as quickly as possible. After a week of silence, finance companies would send us what was called a "ratebook". This was typically an Excel spreadsheet with over 10,000 rows, each representing their "rates" for every available variant of every different make and model. The data in these ratebooks would give us early indicators of what would be competitive this quarter. Spotting the trends was vital, otherwise we could end up without the available vehicles we needed to create competitive deals. If none of this seems relevant, let me explain why it is.

A big part of my job was going through the tens of thousands of cells in these ratebooks and spotting the patterns. If I got It wrong, we could end up with the wrong strategy for the rest of the quarter. Once I spotted a trend, I had to be sure. I kept pages of notes, and wrote down every quote reference number and every discount agreed with every supplier. This meant that if I got it wrong, I could trace back the trail that had led me to an error in judgement. Mistakes happened, but with a good data trail, we could identify them, update our strategy, and carry on.

So a big part of my role was spotting patterns. In fact, I was so good at it, some of the largest vehicle dealerships in the UK would regularly use me as a sounding board to talk through their own strategies for the quarter, despite the fact I was only in my mid-20s.

Without realising it, I was doing the exact same thing during my research on male mental health. I consumed studies quickly, spotted some interesting patterns, and then I tested whether those patterns were real by digging into more detail. Pretty quickly, I could see strong patterns emerging. Specifically, the risk factors that seemed to keep coming up around suicide in men were:

- Poor physical health
- Low socioeconomic status
- Lack of security
- Impulsiveness
- Lack of purpose

Suicide is an enormously complicated issue and there is no single cause or risk factor for suicide. Of course, there are many other factors that aren't listed here, which I don't even have a chance to mention in this book. Sometimes people die from suicide with no signs of suicidal ideation at all, and it is a complete surprise to their friends and loved ones. But what interested me about the above risk factors is that they seemed like things that could potentially be addressed with the right support.

By the end of December 2019, it was 6 months since I had heard the news about Brad, and I had just finished the first version of a framework based on the list above. It was a framework full of proactive, preventative, and practical things I could do.

To protect myself from poor physical health, I researched and designed a lifestyle focussed on testosterone-boosting activities. I called this part of the Framework "**Looking After Body & Mind**". To protect myself from the risk of insecurity, I researched and built practical routines into my life to give me more financial and relationship security. I called this "**Protecting the Cave**". To remind me to take breaks from work, and avoid distracting and addictive things, I researched and began to understand dopamine, and how to regulate it. I called this "**Having Adventures**".

To ensure I kept making progress towards my life goals, I took the goal setting tricks I had learned from managing and coaching my successful sales team (mainly of young men) and started applying them to my life. I called this "**Achieving Recognition**". And to protect myself from a life that lacked purpose, I started to talk to other men about what purpose meant to them, and where they got it from. Eventually, this became known as "**Able to Serve**".

The reason for the names is I wanted to have 5 clear "dimensions" that I could balance to keep myself happy and healthy. And I wanted to fit them into the acronym "ALPHA" because I thought it sounded cool. Years later, this is now known as **The ALPHA Framework**, which I'll share in the next 5 parts of this book. At no point did I ever think that anyone else besides me would ever use this Framework, let alone professionals that work with mental health charities, emergency services, and NHS Trusts.

I hoped at the time that by understanding some of the factors that were associated with suicide in men, I could I could reduce the risk of my mum receiving terrible news, like Jenny did.

Once I started using the Framework, I quickly became much happier and healthier. My life was more structured, balanced, and purposeful. For me personally, The ALPHA Framework provided me with some simple principles to understand myself, make better decisions, and bounce back quicker when I had challenges. It also helped me to communicate when I had issues in my life, and identify the support I needed.

But I never thought that anyone else would want to use it.

I was wrong.

Pretty soon, other men I knew started asking me what I'd started doing differently. When I shared with them what I had learned about testosterone, hormones, and lifestyle, they were often as interested as I was. My research time started being replaced with calls and Zoom meetings with men who wanted to keep up with what I was learning and what I was doing. Some of the men I shared the Framework with started using it to plan their schedule, balancing the time between the different Dimensions.

I had always heard that men are reluctant to talk about mental health, but I found the opposite. When I started sharing relevant and interesting information about measurable things – testosterone, goals, money, for example – men were extremely open to talking to me about their experiences and how it was relevant to their mental health. Conversations regularly lasted hours at a time, and we spoke about everything from what made us feel down, to what stresses us out, and what to do about it all.

These conversations were quite natural for me. Alongside pattern spotting, another big part of my job at the time was helping my relatively young team to understand the complexities of financial regulation, bank lending criteria, and the different vehicle specifications. I did this via a mixture of coaching and training. To me, coaching is simply a set of tools to help others to get clarity on their goals, identify the reasons they haven't achieved those goals, and motivate them to take action. Training is delivering the information and skills that people may need in order to achieve those goals.

While it was fun to share what I had learned about male mental health with other men, it was even more enjoyable to mix in some coaching techniques to motivate them to make some positive lifestyle changes and make use of this new information. The conversations were light-hearted and the early results were extremely positive.

Then, in February 2020, I received a call from a man I will never forget. Christopher.

Christopher explained that I had helped his friend, and he wanted the same support. Christopher had been out of work for 2 years, was very depressed, and was having thoughts about ending his life. I told Christopher that I would love to help him, but if he was having thoughts about suicide, he should be talking to a therapist, not to me. I made him aware that all I was doing was sharing publicly available information with men, along with some coaching techniques to help them make positive life changes. But I wasn't a therapist and this wasn't therapy.

Christopher said he understood that, but he wasn't looking for therapy. He was already in talking therapy, and what he wanted was the kind of accountability and practical suggestions that I had given his friend. Christopher and I agreed to have a short check-in phone call every day for a few weeks to see whether it helped, but he had to stay in talking therapy and call support (like the NHS or Samaritans) if his thoughts became overwhelming. He wanted to pay something for the coaching, as he was used to paying for talking therapy. I donated what he paid me to The OLLIE Foundation, as per my promise to Jenny.

On our third daily check-in call, Christopher told me that *"yesterday was the first day in months"* that he hadn't had any thoughts about suicide. On our tenth daily check-in call, Christopher said that *"yesterday was the first day in years"* that he didn't feel depressed. At the end of the 12 weeks we worked together, he had gone from having no paid work in 2 years, to landing 2 jobs in Netflix productions, and 1 serious acting role in a BBC drama. I was enormously proud of his accomplishments, and so was he.

Christopher was the first man who ever shared with me that he was having thoughts about suicide, but many men have since. I don't believe that his situation improved just by talking to me; it was because of the specific changes that Christopher was prepared to make. In part 2, I will share Christopher's journey in more detail when we explore the science of Achieving Recognition, and how he changed the way he set and pursued his goals.

Wind the clock forwards a few years, and I was still setting time aside to research male mental health and being recommended to other men who wanted to understand themselves better, and make positive life changes. In 2022, I started to receive occasional calls from charities and mental health professionals, who had heard positive things from men who were using The ALPHA Framework. I always took the time to talk them through my Framework, the science behind the different Dimensions, and the practical steps that were in the Framework. I had been constantly revising and updating it, based on the experiences of the men I had worked with, and it was now very different to the early versions. All that remained the same was the name of the Framework and the names of the individual Dimensions.

Some of the professionals I spoke to found the information useful, and recommended me to speak to organisations they worked with. Before I knew it, I was delivering talks to mental health charities, psychotherapists, and suicide prevention charities. Many of which were extremely open to my experience and wanted the opportunity to know what sort of support was working for men. I was able to provide the sources from my research in case they wanted to study the subject further. We swapped ideas and learned from one another.

Without any outreach, marketing, or advertising, I was invited to work with different organisations around the world. At the point of writing this, I have delivered training to psychotherapists, counsellors, and suicide prevention trainers; and talks to police officers, firefighters, and NHS doctors. I've been flown to other continents to speak on stages at conferences and corporate events, sharing my interpretation of scientific studies, turning my experience into workshops with practical takeaways.

The reason I am sharing this part of the story is — just as I made clear to Christopher — I have never tried to position myself as an expert on generalised mental health. I am just a man who has a lot of experience working with men in crisis and can explain how to support them in a way that is inclusive, engaging, and effective. I attend all the courses and training I need to stay informed and ensure safe practice, but I am still not a medical doctor, psychotherapist, or endocrinologist. And I have no intention to ever become any of these. They are all enormously important roles, but they are not my role. My role is to engage with men, equip them with practical tools, and to share what is working in my coaching practice with anyone who wants to support the men in their life or workplace.

The approach I take in this book is not an *alternative* to professional support like medication or talking therapies; but likewise, such professional support should never be seen as an alternative to necessary lifestyle changes. What's needed is a balanced approach where treatments (medicinal and/or therapeutic) are available when needed, but preventative strategies are also provided to reduce the risk of us needing those treatments. Ultimately, every life matters and we should leave no tool unused if it means we can save the men we care about dying from largely preventable killers – like suicide and heart disease.

And if you're with me so far, let me tell you how I have designed this book to be as useful as possible to you.

How to use this book

This book is divided into 8 parts.

Parts 2 to 6 explore the 5 Dimensions of The ALPHA Framework.

In **Part 2: Achieving Recognition**, we will explore a concept called "*socioeconomic status*", and we'll identify a biological mechanism that could explain why low socioeconomic status is associated with depression and suicide rates in men. I'll then share how I believe men can protect themselves against this, by changing the way they set and pursue their goals.

In **Part 3: Looking After Body & Mind**, I will go into more detail as to why low testosterone is linked to all the biggest killers of men, and what we can do about it. I'll also explain why testosterone levels in men are constantly declining and list lifestyle changes that can quickly, naturally, and significantly improve testosterone levels in the men we care about.

In **Part 4: Protecting the Cave**, we will explore the links between financial security, relationship security, and male mental health. We'll explore the evidence from an individual level all the way to large studies, including data from multiple countries. I'll share some of the nuances that are often overlooked when it comes to supporting men and show you how to turn this information into straightforward steps.

In **Part 5: Having Adventures**, we will explore the balancing act of dopamine in our brain, and how certain substances and behaviours cause changes in our brain that undermine discipline and make us more impulsive – a risk factor in both addiction and suicide. I'll also share tools to help us to identify when life is interfering with our dopamine system, when to make changes, and what help and support is out there.

In **Part 6: Able to Serve**, we will look at why the current approach to mental health might not be as effective for men as it is for women, focussing on a missing key aspect that has the potential to engage men and give them a real reason to live, despite the difficulties they may be facing. I'll then share some practical tools that we can all use to help the men we care about to feel more useful.

Each of these parts will start with a list of the specific signs of stress that I look for when I am supporting men. These are not clinical diagnosis tools, they are just patterns I see regularly that help me to understand which Dimensions might be out of balance in a man's life. If you are short on time, they should also help you to focus on the parts of the book that are most relevant to you.

Then each section includes a "story" chapter, focussing on the experiences of a man I have worked with. I've changed any personal details, but included simplified (and realistic) transcripts of me completing a coaching exercise with them, so you can follow the natural flow of the conversations. I'm aware that these are not "normal" conversations. Outside of this specific coaching exercise, no one talks like this, so please don't feel the need to try to replicate it. The purpose of these chapters is not to inspire you to imitate this exercise, it's to give you an insight into the ways that men are thinking about their problems, and the practical solutions they are looking for. I hope they'll make you feel you can talk to men about some of the ideas shared in these transcripts. This creates a "hook" that's often needed to engage men in supportive conversations.

As I mentioned earlier, research is where all this started, and it forms the foundation of every Dimension I've devised to create The ALPHA Framework. So after the "story" of each part, we will delve into the science of each Dimension over 5 separate chapters. The purpose of the "science" chapters is to explain the relevance of each Dimension of The ALPHA Framework, and why the strategies may be effective. Reading the research yourself will help you understand with much greater depth how I arrived at my conclusions. I've tried to include all the references I can in case you want to do your own research or fact-check what I am saying, but I've added them as footnotes so they don't interfere too much with the flow of the book (I promise, the "science" sections are fascinating to read and I've included as little jargon as possible!).

After the "science" sections, I will leave you with specific "strategies" for each Dimension. Not all of them will be appropriate (or even possible) for your situation. It depends on your relationship to and with him, whether you are talking at the moment, how much time you have, and about a million other factors unique to you. You might also find yourself in a situation where you think the strategies could work, but you know you're not the right person to use them. In this case, the bravest thing you can do is to involve the right people. Hopefully this book will give you the information (and reference material) you need to involve the right people at the right time.

You'll see that the "signs of stress" and the titles of the "strategies" are phrased as if we're speaking directly to him. That's intentional. It means you can, if it feels appropriate, show him pages from the book and let him tell you which ones apply to his situation. I do this all the time in coaching, and many people who've attended my workshops have done the same — handing The ALPHA Framework workbook to someone and asking, "Are any of these relevant right now?" This can sometimes open the door to a direct and authentic conversation. If you would like a single page that lists all the signs of stress and strategies in one place, see *The ALPHA Framework: Quick Reference Guide* at the back of this book.

But all this is only useful if you can actually have a supportive conversation with him. In **Part 8: How to Talk to Him** I will pull together everything we've learned and offer my best advice for having supporting conversations with men and boys. I will show why the best-intentioned conversations can often result in a "shutdown" where he doesn't want to open up, followed by a 3-step strategy that I believe is more inclusive, engaging, and effective for men. I'll share example conversations so you can see how the strategy works in reality, and we'll tackle topics that range from suicide to dangerous driving and even getting boys (and men) to help with household chores. This part finishes with some simple word swaps that can help you to bridge the barriers with the males in your work, life, and home.

And if this book helps prevent the loss of even 1 man like Brad, and spares just 1 person from the pain that Jenny endured, then every hour of research, every day spent writing, every penny spent on printing – and your investment in reading it – will have been worth it.

ENDNOTES

1. If you're reading my footnotes, you'll see that each reference starts with an 'R' number. That matches a specific row in the spreadsheet containing all my sources—around 1,500 at the time of publishing. You can download the full spreadsheet at TheMensCoach.co.uk/science. The publisher and I decided to keep these 'R' numbers in to make it easier for you to explore the references and do your own research if you'd like to.
2. R164: Samaritans (Accessed 2025). "Latest suicide data." samaritans.org.
3. R167: H Godfrey (2021). "London buses to double passenger capacity from Monday." CityAM.
4. R743: S Bennett et al. (2023). "Male suicide and barriers to accessing professional support: a qualitative thematic analysis." Current Psychology.
5. TheOllieFoundation.org
6. R165: GOVUK (2017). "Chapter 2: major causes of death and how they have changed." GOV.UK.
7. I'm afraid I don't know which studies I first found this in, but I've included two similar studies as sources to back up the figures I make reference to.
8. R229: V Čulić (2013). "Daylight saving time transitions and acute myocardial infarction." The Journal of Biological and Medical Rhythm Research.
9. R228: I Kirchberger (2015). "Are daylight saving time transitions associated with changes in myocardial infarction incidence? Results from the German MONICA/KORA Myocardial Infarction Registry." BMC Public Health.
10. R128: P Patel et al. (2018). "Impaired sleep is associated with low testosterone in us adult males: results from the national health and nutrition survey." Fertility and Sterility.

11 R561: C M Swartz et al. (1987). "Low serum testosterone and myocardial infarction in geriatric male inpatients." Journal of the American Geriatrics Society.
12 R142: T Goodale et al. (2017). "Testosterone and the heart." Methodist Debakey Cardiovasc Journal.
13 R604: R Leproult et al. (2011). "Effect of 1 week of sleep restriction on testosterone levels in young healthy men." JAMA.
14 R1204: S Duke et al. (2014). "Testosterone and its effects on human male adolescent mood and behavior: A systematic review." Journal of Adolescent Health.
15 R1205: S Geniole et al. (2020). "Is testosterone linked to human aggression? A meta-analytic examination of the relationship between baseline, dynamic, and manipulated testosterone on human aggression." Hormones and Behavior.
16 R1129: J Carré et al. (2018). "Testosterone and human behavior: the role of individual and contextual variables." Current Opinion in Psychology.
17 R1207: Jeremy Aikey et al. (2002). "Testosterone rapidly reduces anxiety in male house mice (mus musculus)." Hormones and Behavior.
18 R1208: J Hodosy et al. (2012). "The anxiolytic effect of testosterone in the rat is mediated via the androgen receptor." Pharmacology Biochemistry and Behavior.
19 R1151: D Rubinow et al. (2005). "Testosterone suppression of CRH-stimulated cortisol in men." Neuropsychopharmacology.
20 R126: J Johnson et al. (2013). "The effect of testosterone levels on mood in men: A review." Psychosomatics.
21 In this book, when I talk about testosterone, I am generally talking about what is often called 'total' or 'serum' testosterone. This is the amount of testosterone circulating in the blood, some of which is active but most of which is bound to proteins. Total testosterone is only a single measurement of male hormonal health, but I believe it's more useful (and interesting) than most people know!
22 R270: Schweiger, Ulrich et al. (1999). "Testosterone, gonadotropin, and cortisol secretion in male patients with major depression." Psychosomatic Medicine.
23 R133: R McIntyre et al. (2006). "Calculated bioavailable testosterone levels and depression in middle-aged men." Psychoneuroendocrinology.
24 R552: O P Almeida et al. (2008). "Low free testosterone concentration as a potentially treatable cause of depressive symptoms in older men." JAMA Psychiatry.
25 R839: M M Shores et al. (2005). "Low testosterone levels predict incident depressive illness in older men: effects of age and medical morbidity." The Journal of Clinical Psychiatry.
26 R122: A Walther et al. (2019). "Association of testosterone treatment with alleviation of depressive symptoms in men: A systematic review and meta-analysis." JAMA Psychiatry.
27 R556: T G Travison et al. (2017). "Harmonized reference ranges for circulating testosterone levels in men of four cohort studies in the United States and Europe." The Journal of Clinical Endocrinology & Metabolism.
28 R133: R McIntyre et al. (2006). "Calculated bioavailable testosterone levels and depression in middle-aged men." Psychoneuroendocrinology.
29 R1106: J Tripodianakis, M Markianos et al. (2007). "Gonadal axis hormones in psychiatric male patients after a suicide attempt." European Archives of Psychiatry and Clinical Neuroscience.

30   R1105: M Markianos, J Tripodianakis et al. (2009). "Suicide attempt by jumping: A study of gonadal axis hormones in male suicide attempters versus men who fell by accident." Psychiatry Research.

31   R1111: L Sher et al. (2021). "The effect of oral dexamethasone administration on testosterone levels in combat veterans with or without a history of suicide attempt." Journal of Psychiatric Research.

32   R842: B Roland et al. (1986). "Proposed relation of testosterone levels to male suicides and sudden deaths." Psychological Reports.

33   Another problem with the Roland et al. (1986) study is that it appears to have completely confused testosterone units. The study claims that all measurements are ng/mL, but clearly is using ng/dL. You can see this is a mistake by looking at the reference range that they include in the article ("300 to 1,000 ng/mL", which should be 300 to 1,000 ng/dL). This may explain why the team who carried out the study misinterpreted their own findings – they just weren't familiar enough with testosterone measurements to spot an obvious mistake. Unfortunately, the mistake was also missed by the publisher and at least 3 peer reviewed articles that have cited it since. To my knowledge, I am the only person who has spotted this. But get in contact if you disagree.

34   An example of an article that uses the Roland et al. (1986) study as an argument that high testosterone may be associated with risk of suicide is R1144: L Sher (2013). "High and low testosterone levels may be associated with suicidal behavior in young and older men, respectively." Australian & New Zealand Journal of Psychiatry. However the lead author's later work with male military veterans found that higher testosterone levels were not associated with suicide; lower levels were.

35   Besides the Roland et al. (1986) study, the other research often used to support the idea that higher testosterone is linked to increased suicide in men tends to come from studies on men with bipolar disorder or from J. Zhang et al. (2015). In men with bipolar disorder, higher testosterone has been associated with suicide, which is an important finding. But we can't presume this applies to men without bipolar, because bipolar is linked with changes in both stress hormones and sex hormones. The J. Zhang et al. (2015) study is also often cited, but their control group only had an average testosterone level of 14.4 nmol/L (which makes me wonder whether they were experiencing other health issues); the article confused testosterone units at one stage (similar to issues in the Roland et al. study); and once they accounted for other factors, the link between higher testosterone and suicide risk wasn't statistically significant. Personally, I think this can be a bit of a distraction from the studies showing much lower testosterone levels in men who think about, attempt, or die from suicide. My goal with this footnote is not to discredit any important work, but to explain that I have read the counter-argument in detail and think it can be interpreted without jumping to the conclusion that higher testosterone is linked to suicide in men. For reference, in case you'd like to read it: R1135: J Zhang et al (2015). "Testosterone differs between suicide attempters and community controls in men and women of China." Physiology & Behavior.

36   R165: GOV.UK (2017). "Chapter 2: major causes of death and how they have changed." GOV.UK.

37 R1480: B Yeap et al. (2024). "Associations of testosterone and related hormones with all-cause and cardiovascular mortality and incident cardiovascular disease in men: individual participant data meta-analyses." Annals of Internal Medicine.
38 R561: C Swartz et al. (1987). "Low serum testosterone and myocardial infarction in geriatric male inpatients." Journal of the American Geriatrics Society.
39 R142: T Goodale et al. (2017). "Testosterone and the heart." Methodist Debakey Cardiovascular Journal.
40 R165: GOV.UK (2017). "Chapter 2: major causes of death and how they have changed." GOV.UK.
41 R557: Prostate Cancer UK (2023). "About Prostate Cancer." prostatecanceruk.org.
42 R1512: J Lillard et al. (2022). "Racial disparities in Black men with prostate cancer: A literature review." Cancer.
43 R117: J Park et al. (2016). "Low testosterone level is an independent risk factor for high-grade prostate cancer detection at biopsy." BJU International.
44 R301: X Xu et al. (2018). "Dynamic patterns of testosterone levels in individuals and risk of prostate cancer among hypogonadal men: a longitudinal study." The Journal of Urology.
45 I am also aware that men with "unusually low levels of testosterone" are at a 20% lower risk of developing prostate cancer than those with a normal level, but given how that could impact a man's overall quality of life, I wouldn't recommend that a man aims for a low level when a higher level may be many times more protective. Interestingly, this large study of 19,000 men also found that when men with the lowest levels of testosterone develop prostate cancer, it is 65% more likely to be aggressive: R1212: The National Cancer Research Institute (NCRI) (2017). "Low testosterone levels are linked to reduced risk of prostate cancer." cancerresearchuk.org.
46 R912: A Morgentaler et al. (1996). "Occult prostate cancer in men with low serum testosterone levels." JAMA.
47 R864: M Ribeiro et al. (1997). "Low serum testosterone and a younger age predict for a poor outcome in metastatic prostate cancer." American Journal of Clinical Oncology.
48 R165: GOV.UK (2017). "Chapter 2: major causes of death and how they have changed." GOV.UK.
49 R836: A Zonderman et al. (2005). "Predicting Alzheimer's disease in the Baltimore longitudinal study of aging." Journal of Geriatric Psychiatry and Neurology.
50 R1369: B Yeap & L Flicker (2022). "Testosterone, cognitive decline and dementia in ageing men." Reviews in Endocrine and Metabolic Disorders.
51 R1292: M Muehlenbein et al. (2022). "Lower testosterone levels are associated with higher risk of death in men." Evolution, Medicine, and Public Health.
52 R1165: E Barrett-Connor (2012). "The Rancho Bernardo Study: 40 years studying why women have less heart disease than men and how diabetes modifies women's usual cardiac protection." Global Heart.
53 All the labs and organisations I have referenced draw the upper limit of "normal" around 30 nmol/L.

PART 2:

ACHIEVING RECOGNITION

"A musician must make music, an artist must paint, a poet must write, if he is to be ultimately at peace with himself. What a man can be, he must be."

– Abraham Maslow

Achieving Recognition	
Signs of stress	-Feeling *stuck* or *unsuccessful* -Lack of written goals -Outcome-based goals -Comparison with others -Loss of social status (redundancy, retirement)

Christopher's story

"We're going to do a coaching exercise," I told Christopher over a Zoom call. He leaned back in his seat in a way that told me he was feeling a little uncomfortable. And that was OK. I told him he and I were going to role-play a phone call together, and there were some rules to follow.

"Rule number one," I said. "This call is taking place one year from today. And so if you want to tell me about all the incredible things you have achieved, you need to tell me what you *have done*, not what you are *planning to do*."

Christopher nodded his head solemnly.

"Rule number two: The call doesn't end until I say: 'Anyway, I've got to go but it was great talking to you, Christopher, BEEP.' It will feel like I'm ending the Zoom call, but I'm not, I'm just ending the coaching exercise.

"And rule number three: the first words you're going to say are going to be: '*Holy shit, Ryan, my life is so good right now, I just called to tell you all about it.*' Don't try to take notes. Don't think. Nothing that you say is wrong. Nothing is embarrassing."

With Christopher's agreement, we began.

Christopher's Future Call

Ryan: Ring-ring! Ring-ring! Ah, Christopher. I wasn't expecting your call – how are you doing?

Christopher: Holy crap, man. My life is so good. I've had such a good year. I just wanted to tell you about it...

[Christopher paused for a moment as his eyes filled with tears. He drew a breath and carried on.]

Ryan: Go on, man. What have you been up to?

Christopher: I landed a big role in a drama series... Yeah, I'm in New Zealand right now. We're filming these amazing scenes. I wish you could see it, man. And things back home are so much better. I've got a brand-new agent now. She's got real sway. She can find me opportunities and get me into the big leagues.

[Christopher carried on, naming all the brilliant achievements of the previous year. For each achievement, I asked him what obstacles he had to overcome. Once I was confident that he was ready, I asked him 5 important coaching questions that I wanted him to answer.]

Ryan: Cast your mind back to when we had that very first Zoom call together one year ago... At the time, what was the main thing that was holding you back?

Christopher: At the time... I was having to turn down unpaid work. Last year, I was working with this agent... She was great at her job, but she didn't want me to "*cheapen my brand*" by working in small productions. When I started turning down those small gigs, everything changed. The stage time practically disappeared... so did the practice... so did the time with my friends... A few weeks later I began to feel down. And a few months later I started thinking about ending it all. I've never actually connected those things until this conversation.

Ryan: What did you do to overcome the lack of unpaid work?

Christopher: I decided I was going to act at every opportunity, even if I didn't get paid. Even if my agent didn't like it. I realised that, for me, acting is not just a job, it's my passion. I realised that the only way to be true to myself... was to follow my heart. And my heart led me onto the stages with the best stories... My heart led me to some of the most meaningful performances of my life. Because it wasn't ever about the money, it was about being the man that I needed to be. I had to prove I could do it. For me, the only way to stop thinking about suicide was to build the life I actually wanted to live. Everything else was just plastering over the cracks.

Ryan: Well done, Christopher. You've had an amazing year, but I want to know: what has been the single best thing you've done all year?

Christopher: I invited my dad on set. It was such a proud moment, man. When he saw how hard I had worked, and how much I love the work, he finally got it. There was this moment where it felt like we finally understood each other. A moment where he finally saw me as a capable man.

Ryan: If I had a time machine, and you could send a message back in time to be delivered to Christopher at the end of his first coaching session one year ago, what would you say to him? What did he need to hear at the time?

Christopher: ... I would say to him... "*Get back on the bloody stage. Get back on set, lad. It's where you need to be. Somewhere along the lines, you lost sight of that. It's not the contract that makes you an actor. It's not the bloody money, or the bloody agent, or even the fans. It's the acting. It's your love for your craft. It's your dedication to understanding your character. Don't you ever forget that. You are an actor. Now go and be one!"*

Ryan: It's been an absolute honour seeing what you've achieved over the past year, Christopher, but I want to know... Cast your mind back to that first coaching session we had a year ago. When you left the coaching call, what was the very first thing you did that got this amazing year off to a great start?

Christopher: I opened a list of casting directors' emails and I began contacting them. This bloody list had sat on my laptop for over a year. It was just too daunting a task to start. I wasn't only scared that I might fail; I was scared that I might actually succeed. I was scared to find out whether it could actually happen. But email by email, day by day, audition by audition, I built this career with my bare hands. I made this happen. The first thing I did a year ago today... Was to send my first email to a casting director.

Ryan: Well done, man. Well, you've had an amazing year and it's been my honour to watch you achieve so much. I know there were times where you made use of the expertise of others – friends, family, your therapist, your mentors – but ultimately *YOU* made this happen. You realised what you really wanted and you went for it. And I want you to know that your dad's proud of you, your friends are proud of you, I'm proud of you, and you should be proud of yourself.

Christopher: Thank you, Ryan.

Ryan: Look, I have to go now, but it was great catching up.

Christopher: Cheers, man.

Ryan: Cheers, Christopher.
BEEP

The coaching exercise ended and Christopher stared into his camera with a new look of determination in his eyes. After a few minutes of silence, he began to speak. "I know what I need to do. Thank you."

After our first coaching call, I set Christopher the challenge of calling me every morning at 7 a.m. and telling me what progress he made yesterday towards his goal of acting at every opportunity. You will recall from when I introduced you to Christopher in the introduction how he secured roles in Netflix and with the BBC. Years later, he is still a professional actor. Many of his biggest roles can be traced back to emails he sent out during those first few weeks of working together — all part of his new way of setting goals for himself.

The first A in ALPHA stands for **Achieving Recognition**. It's about the things men need to do for their sense of success.

Achieving Recognition: The science

The risk is not spread evenly amongst men

Every 10 years in the UK, the Office for National Statistics carries out a census. Every adult has to complete the census, confirming where they live, where they work, how much they earn, and lots of other information. This means that in the UK, a significant amount of social and economic data is collected.

And once you overlay this data with suicide statistics, it tells a very interesting story about men.

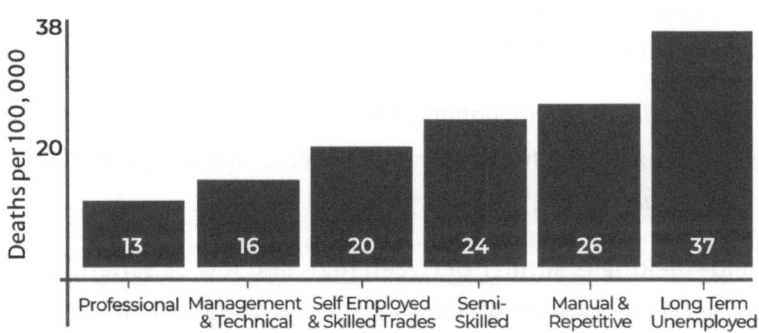

Adapted from R894: Office for National Statistics (2023). "Sociodemographic inequalities in suicides in England and Wales: 2011 to 2021." ons.gov.uk. Grouping based on NS-SEC: 1.1, 1.2 ('Professional'); 2 ('Management & Technical'); 4, 5 ('Self-Employed & Skilled Trades'); 6 ('Semi-Skilled'); 7 ('Manual & Repetitive').

The type of work men do is strongly linked to their suicide risk, with men in manual and repetitive roles being significantly more likely to die from suicide than their immediate managers — even if they work in the same industry.

And it's not just the type of work that predicts risk of suicide and depression in men, so does the area they live in. According to UK suicide prevention charity, Samaritans, *"Men from the lowest social class, living in the most deprived areas, are up to 10 more likely to end their lives by suicide than those in the highest social class from the most affluent areas."* [1]

This means that there is a big disparity of risk between different groups of men *and* the risk of suicide isn't evenly distributed amongst men. In fact, it tends to correlate strongly with a factor known as "socioeconomic status".

Socioeconomic status (SES) refers to our social and economic position in society. Statisticians often place people into SES groups based on the job we do. They do this because how skilled, well-paid, or prestigious our job is usually reflects other factors — such as our income, education, where we live, access to healthcare, and other social factors that are harder to measure but still important. SES therefore represents not just what we earn but also the wider advantages or disadvantages that shape our lives.

Before I began learning about male mental health, I had always heard that the reason men died from suicide at higher rates than women was because they are less likely to reach out for help. But this argument starts to fall apart when you compare different groups of men. In a 2012 report, UK suicide prevention charity Samaritans, advised that:

"While higher educated and higher earning men are more likely to know about therapy and are more likely to know how to get formal help, they are not more likely to reach out for help." [2]

Since help-seeking is similar between high and low SES men, but suicide rates are very different, it seems misguided to suggest that high suicide rates in men are simply a result of them not reaching out for help.

Another common explanation I had frequently heard was how men might lack emotional skills, placing them at higher risk of suicide than women. But that argument, too, falls apart once you compare different groups of men. In the same report, Samaritans went on to suggest that, in order to support men, it might be more useful to focus on the socioeconomic factors that place men at higher risk of suicide *"rather than on less prominent class differences in the emotional skills of men"*.

Many of the majority-male organisations I work with see the same trend in their industry. Like many around the world, the UK construction industry has a high rate of death from suicide: in 2021, over 99% of those who died from suicide in the industry were male. But the risk isn't spread evenly.

Let me show you what I mean using 2021 data.

Classes of construction work	Rate of suicide (per 100, 000)
Professionals & management *Architects, chartered surveyors, engineers*	11
Skilled trades *Bricklayers, carpenters, painters, roofers*	38
Entry-level *Prep, cleaning, and movement of tools, machines and assets in the construction industry**	78
UK male average (the same year, for reference)	16

* The specific role referred to here is elementary construction occupations. For more information, see R695: CareerSmart (2023). "Elementary Construction Occupations." *careersmart.org.uk*.

Adapted from R1023: Office For National Statistics (2024). "Suicides in England and Wales: 2022 registrations." *ons.gov.uk* and R266: The Construction Index (2022). "Construction suicides keep rising." *theconstructionindex.co.uk*.

Mirroring the pattern outside of the construction industry, employment type is related to male suicide rate. While those in manual and repetitive construction roles were nearly 5× more likely to die from suicide than the average UK male, professionals in the same industry were significantly less likely to die from suicide than the average UK male (11 deaths per 100,000, compared with the UK average of 16 per 100,000).

In the words of another Samaritans study:

"The least skilled occupations have higher rates of suicide." [3]

There's also an association between low socioeconomic status and depression in men. In 2019, a study of 18,571 people (8,236 of which were men) used a mental health questionnaire to identify major depression and overlaid the home address of each participant with census data to assess the affluence of their area. The study found that:

"Men living in the most deprived areas were 51% more likely to have depression than those living in areas that were not deprived, but the association between deprivation and [major depression] was not statistically significant in women. [...] This study shows that the residential environment differentially affects men and women, and this needs to be taken into account by mental health policy-makers." [4]

And a study of 23,794 adults in Stockholm found that occupational class was a predictor of future depression, with men in unskilled manual roles being 3× more likely to become depressed than men in higher roles over the next 5 years. Interestingly, this link between occupation type and depression was not seen in women. [5]

It seems pretty evident that socioeconomic status is particularly important for male mental health, especially when it comes to protecting against depression and suicide.

I am sure there are many complicated and confounding factors behind this, but there's one in particular we are going to explore. It starts with understanding how we are the only animal that has been known to ever deliberately take its own life. Yes, other animals have been found to put themselves at risk of harm for the benefit of their group, and some have been found to harm themselves. But even in our closest relatives – chimpanzees and bonobos – there has not been any evidence of deliberate intention to end their own lives. Suicide, it seems, is a uniquely human behaviour. This would suggest there is something unique in our biology that allows for suicide, which no other animals seem to have. [6]

So let's start there, with an exploration of our biology.

Serotonin: The "good news" neurotransmitter

Your body is full of chemical messengers. In your blood they're called hormones; in your brain they're called neurotransmitters. These chemical messengers play a crucial role in almost every process in your brain and body.

When it comes to mental health, there is one chemical messenger that plays an especially important role: serotonin, which is both a neurotransmitter and a hormone. While most of the serotonin you make is produced in the gut to regulate digestion, the serotonin in your brain plays a vital role in positive mental health.

In your brain, serotonin protects you from stress, helps you to think long term, and is associated with positive mental health and emotions. Low levels of serotonin make us more vulnerable to stress, and are associated with depression, violent and impulsive behaviour, and – in humans – suicide. [7][8]

In 1994, a 12-month study of suicide attempters found that those with below-average levels of brain serotonin were 2.4× more likely to die from suicide over the study period than those with above average levels. [9]

Then, in 2005, 15 male suicide attempters who arrived at the Karolinska Hospital in Sweden were assessed using 2 questionnaires, plus their brain serotonin levels. The questionnaires were the Beck's Suicide Intent Scale (SIS) and the Beck Hopelessness Scale (BHS) – both designed to assess risk of suicide. The men were followed up for 2 years.

Sadly, 5 of the men died from suicide during the study period. The study found that while neither of the questionnaires had predicted who would go on to take their own lives, the serotonin levels had. The men with low serotonin levels at the beginning of the study were the ones who died over the next 2 years. The study concluded: *"In high suicide risk hospitalised male psychiatric patients [serotonin levels] may be a better predictor of early suicide after attempted suicide than SIS or BHS."* [10]

And in 2009, a review published in the *Oxford Textbook of Suicidology and Suicide Prevention* stated that the 2 most reliable biological predictors of future suicide risk appear to be:

1. low levels of brain serotonin, and
2. stress hormone imbalances.

Each of these factors was associated with *"about 4.5-fold greater risk of suicide."* Fundamentally, these 2 things happening at the same time would be particularly dangerous. [11]

So far we've explored how men with low socioeconomic status are at increased risk of suicide and depression. And we've looked at how depression and suicide appear to be linked to low serotonin levels. Next I want to show you how these things appear to be connected.

Serotonin: How males track social status

Besides promoting positive mental health, serotonin also plays another role, though it's less well known: in male primates, serotonin seems to keep track of their place within social hierarchies.

Studies on different types of primates have found that, in males, serotonin increases and decreases in line with their social status. Studies of squirrel monkeys show that the most senior male seems to have serotonin levels around 40% higher than the next social rank. And they, in turn, have serotonin levels about 20% higher than the next rank of males. The difference between males is even more pronounced in vervet monkeys. In this species, the highest ranking male has serotonin levels around 80% higher than the other members of his group. [12]

These high levels of serotonin return to normal when the high-ranking males are separated from their male supporters. By removing "subordinate males" from the group, researchers can reduce serotonin levels in high-ranking male primates back to normal levels, even when the females remain. These serotonin levels appear to be a method of monitoring social status against other males.

Which made me wonder: Do *human* males have a similar mechanism built into their biology? Do their serotonin levels rise when their social status increases, and fall when it is reduced?

Our societies are a lot more complicated than the monkey societies I have previously described. Unlike other primates, there are almost infinite ways we can measure ourselves — from skill and rank to income and wealth.

One aspect that makes our social rank so tricky to determine is its fluidity. After all, at the end of my working day, I might walk away from a job where I am the most junior member of the team and head to my football practice, where I am the club captain.

But the perception of rank is built into human organisations. Take work as an example, where we are often placed into an 'organisational chart' and report to a manager — or have people report to us. We feel social rank when we are physically nervous talking to a CEO in the boardroom or to our university professor after class. It also happens in our social lives, like when you join a club or, if you go to an American university, a fraternity. A small American study of young men found that fraternity officers had 25% higher levels of serotonin than those who saw them as leaders. [13]

There is a line of thought that *socioeconomic status* is the closest measure we have to social rank. This made me wonder whether serotonin levels in human males rise with higher socioeconomic status. Turns out, I wasn't the first person to ask that question... [14]

In 2000, researchers carried out an experiment on 270 adults to answer this question. They looked at how each participant reacted to a drug that boosts serotonin activity (the drug was *fenfluramine*), and used family income and education level to assess socioeconomic status. They found that both men and women with lower socioeconomic status had a weaker response to the drug—meaning their brains didn't seem to produce as much serotonin as you might expect. This couldn't be explained by factors like age, gender, or body size. [15]

Over the following years, similar studies had very similar findings. But they also found that the affluence of our neighbourhood impacts brain serotonin more than other social factors such as income or education level. [16]

Given that living in an affluent area positively impacts serotonin and low serotonin is linked with suicide, you can probably see why Samaritans found that:

"Men who are less well-off and living in the most deprived areas are up to 10 times more likely to die by suicide than more well-off men from affluent areas." [17]

And while I am focussing on the mental health inequality associated with social class in men, there's also strong evidence that socioeconomic status plays a large role in physical health too. In an old – but famous – study, researchers followed 11,678 male civil servants for 10 years and found that social status (measured by employment grade and car ownership, back when cars were less common) was a strong predictor of life expectancy. Men in the lowest employment grade who didn't own a car were over 4× more likely to die (from any cause, not necessarily suicide) during the study period, compared to those in the highest grade who owned a car. Known risk factors – smoking, blood cholesterol, blood pressure, and insulin resistance – could not explain the disparity in risk. The patterns remained consistent even in men who reported no health issues at the beginning of the study. [18]

When the study was repeated 20 years later, researchers found the same thing: lower socioeconomic status predicted worse physical health. Despite how far we had come medically in 2 decades, the gap between different social classes wasn't closing for physical health, any more than mental health. [19]

The final interesting pattern I spotted regarding rank was to do with loss of status in the workplace. I work with many types of organisations that have a fixed hierarchy, like emergency service providers. It is well known within these organisations that when men lose their rank, it can have a catastrophic impact on their mental health. This is not only in the case of a demotion or suspension; it can also be in the case of a retirement. In either case, losing the title seems to mean much more than losing a job; he has also lost his associated protective social status.

Let's recap:

- Low socioeconomic status predicts increased future risk of depression and suicide in men.

- Low brain serotonin predicts increased future risk of depression and suicide.
- In many primate species, serotonin levels in males are directly linked to social status.
- We appear to be one of those species.

Am I suggesting that there is nothing we can do, and that men with lower socioeconomic status are doomed to worse mental and physical health?

Absolutely not.

I wanted to share these studies on social status and serotonin because I am always surprised that they aren't a major part of the conversation about male mental health, even though the evidence looks pretty compelling.

However, I believe that the link between social status and serotonin may actually be a byproduct of something else. From working directly with men, I've come to suspect that it's not socioeconomic status itself that affects mental health, but a man's *sense of success*. Socioeconomic factors — like a high rank at work or living in an affluent area - might make some men feel more successful, but not all men. And for many men - especially those with lower SES - the challenge is that there are simply more barriers standing between them and their sense of success. [20]

Sense of success: The 2 factors that make it

Your sense of success depends on 2 main factors:

1. Your *definition* of success
2. How far you feel from it

When I started working with Christoper, his definition of success was *being a professional actor*. But since he wasn't one, this lack of alignment left him feeling unsuccessful - and his lack of progress made him feel stuck.

I asked him, "Once you are a professional actor, how will you spend your time?" He told me that he will act at every opportunity, even if he doesn't get paid. If there were no big roles, he would do small ones. If there were no small ones, he would perform monologues to his camera and post them online. Ironically, this was not only how he imagined successful actors spent their time, but it was also completely within his control.

Over time, Christopher redefined what success meant to him:

1. Definition of success: act at every opportunity
2. How far away he felt from it: he could start doing it today

By shifting his definition to something he could control, Christopher closed the gap between who he was and who he wanted to be. And once he closed that gap, his mental health improved significantly — even though his socioeconomic status hadn't changed at all.

I regularly work with men who may appear successful to others, but don't feel successful inside. And likewise with men who do not need a prestigious job, car, or house to feel successful. And why should they?

So far as I know, there is no research into a man's sense of success impacting his brain serotonin levels, but there are little clues to support this notion.

In 2021, an American study set out to understand whether women and men needed different support after a suicide attempt. They interviewed 50 military veterans to find out what had worked for them. (Military veterans are often the participants of studies on suicide because they are known to be at higher risk.) The study's conclusion:

"Findings suggest that recovery needs among veterans after a nonfatal suicide attempt vary by gender: women may benefit more from psychoeducational approaches in group settings with other women, whereas men may benefit more from approaches that help them focus on making changes in their lives towards becoming their ideal selves." [21]

If you're happy with me rephrasing this to my approach, it would be something like this:

As part of recovering from a suicide attempt, women may benefit more from understanding and expressing how they feel in group settings with other women, whereas men may benefit more from approaches that help them close the gap between who they are and who they want to be.

My theory is that it's not the socioeconomic status that boosts serotonin levels in men, it's feeling successful. Men with higher socioeconomic status have fewer obstacles to fulfilling their sense of success. By contrast, men with lower socioeconomic status (less job autonomy, less financial control, fewer career options) have more obstacles, often finding themselves stuck in the "gap" between who they are and who they want to be.

Unfortunately, the way that we set goals often adds to this problem.

The way we set goals often makes things worse

The way that many of us have been encouraged to set goals is something like:

1. Decide what you want
2. Break that down into small steps
3. Visualise how achieving your goal will change your life

From now on, I'm going to refer to this method as traditional goal setting. But for many people, this way of setting goals actually makes them feel *less* successful.

The problem with traditional goal setting is that it:

1. Focusses too much on the outcome

When I met Christopher, his goal was to "*be a professional actor*". This is a good example of a bad goal. As soon as he set this goal for himself, he increased the gap between **who he was** and **who he wanted to be**.

In my experience, it's not that men who are depressed don't have goals. Paradoxically, in some instances, their goals are part of the reason they feel depressed. Many of the most depressed men I have worked with had a "vision board" that they looked at every day, with a picture of a house they can't afford, a car they will never drive, and an Oscar they will probably never win. This focus on what they don't have made them less content with their own life and feel less successful.

2. Does not identify the best ways to achieve the goal

Because we tend to set goals for things we haven't done before, it's very likely that we don't actually know how to achieve the goal we have just set. Traditional goal setting does very little to help with this. And so, many men have set extremely specific goals (for example, SMART goals) but have very little idea how to close the gap they have just created in their life. This is like having the exact GPS coordinates but no navigation system to guide you there.

3. Does not identify why you haven't already achieved the goal

When setting a goal, one of the most important questions we can ask ourselves is why we haven't already achieved the goal yet. If you've been on the planet for decades and something hasn't already happened, there's probably a reason for it. Without this insight, we will continue to set goals that are doomed to failure from the start, because we are not addressing the real obstacles in our life.

4. Let's you set goals outside of your control

Back to Christopher's goal of "being a professional actor". One of the issues with this goal is that it relies on other people. He couldn't be a professional actor on his own, it would require someone else to hire him. By setting goals that are beyond our control, our sense of success now depends on luck and other people.

5. Makes it hard to build on your momentum

The other issue with outcome-based goals is that, perhaps contradictorily, they cause a "cliff-edge" situation where motivation is totally lost if the goal is actually achieved. We all know someone who trained regularly for a year to complete a marathon, and then hasn't run since. Or someone who saved for years for a round-the-world adventure, but has never saved a penny since that trip. Outcome-based goals make it hard to build on past successes, meaning we find ourselves always "looking for that next thing" to stay motivated.

In summary, traditional goal setting causes us to set goals that:

1. make us less content with what we have
2. we don't know how to achieve

3. don't address the obstacles we will encounter
4. are outside of our control, and
5. will cause a drop in motivation if we do manage to achieve them

You can probably see why YouGov found that 22% of people who set New Year's resolutions have broken them by 6 January, and GoalsCalling.com states that only 6% of people regularly set and achieve their goals. The way that we have been taught to set goals just doesn't work for most people. [22] [23]

My experience working with hundreds of men on their life goals is that when they learn how to set the *right* goals, their mental health quickly improves. This is the essence of what I mean by Achieving Recognition. It is the Dimension associated with closing the gap between who men are and who they want to be – potentially protecting them from the social factors that put them at risk of suicide.

Achieving Recognition: Strategies

Achieving Recognition is about feeling successful. In this part of the book, we have explored how low socioeconomic status impacts brain serotonin levels in men, and the protective role of goal setting. We can all support the men we care about by first offering them clarity and then accountability around their goals.

❑ Write down life goals

Encourage the men in your life to write down their goals. This goes for everything from the smallest to the most ambitious goals, and it isn't just to aid memory! There is some evidence that once a goal is written down it is about 42% more likely to be completed, compared to simply thinking about it. You can easily support the men you care about by encouraging them to put pen to paper when they mention any of their goals. [24]

This is one of the first things that Christopher and I did together. For years he had lots of goals floating around in his head, but he had never actually sat down and made a list of what he wanted to achieve and then approached it in a structured way. Doing so gave us both a sense of clarity.

❏ Identify obstacles

One of the most powerful questions for supporting others – including men – is "What is the main thing that's holding you back?" I recommend you ask it when anyone shares their goals with you.

This question can cut through the fog and get right to the heart of problems.

When I asked Christopher this question, he told me that his new agent had stopped him from doing "poorly paid" acting work, in case it devalued his brand. He had gone from acting regularly, practising his skills, and spending time with his friends, to sitting at home, waiting for the email inbox to ping with a "big" opportunity.

There is no way I could have known something like that was having such a significant impact on his life, but being asked this question allowed him to take me straight to the root of the problem. This question is such a useful tool to help people identify the obstacles in their own life, which is required for the next steps.

❏ Set weekly goals

Once a goal is written down and obstacles have been identified, it's important to identify an action (however small) that would start to address the obstacles, giving a sense of progress.

Ask the question: "What could you do in the next seven days that would give you a sense of progress towards that goal?" I have found weekly goals are enormously important. Taking weekly action is the difference between having a goal and having a dream.

❏ Weekly goals should be small, effort-based, and wholly within your control

Be mindful of the goals that you hear men set for themselves. By setting the wrong type of goals, men often externalise their sense of success, fail to start, or are vulnerable to being let down by others. By setting the right goals, men can internalise their sense of success, relying less on external factors and luck.

After working with hundreds of men over thousands of separate coaching and accountability calls, I have found that great weekly goals are:

1. small enough to not cause fear or procrastination
2. based on effort (what we put in) not outcome (what we get out), and
3. wholly within our own control

Based on these rules, the goal *"Write 1,000 words of my essay"* becomes *"Open my laptop each morning and type 1 word"* – who could put that off?

"Do well at my job interview" becomes *"Be ready for my job interview"* – focusing on what he can control.

And *"Meet my friend for dinner"* becomes *"Close my laptop at 6 p.m., ready to meet my friend for dinner"*. This way even an unreliable friend can't stop him from achieving his goal.

In Christopher's case, his goal went from *"I will be a professional actor"* (outcome-based) to *"I will act every week, even if I don't get paid for it"* (effort-based). This got him back onto stages and film sets, meeting others in his industry and practising his skills. Suddenly, people saw him as an actor and job offers began to come in again. By not focussing on the outcome, he achieved the outcome that had eluded him for years.

❏ Arrange weekly accountability

It's been found that when a person does the following 3 things, the chances of achieving a goal seem to increase by 76%, compared to simply thinking about it:

1. write down a goal
2. break it down into weekly actions
3. share their weekly progress with others

You may be able to support him with the third step by offering that weekly accountability, or asking him who would be a good source of accountability.

Ask him to pick his own accountability question that you will ask him each week (this ensures you use the words that he finds relevant and motivating). Then pick a regular time to have a phone call. It doesn't need to take more than a few minutes a week.

When I asked Christopher what kind of accountability he would like, he said that each morning when we spoke, I should ask him: *"What did you do yesterday to improve as an actor?"* Once he stopped having thoughts about suicide, we dropped the calls down to each Monday morning.

It's important that when you put accountability questions in place, you both stick to the agreed time and wording. Christopher's words were important because he chose them. The accountability calls would have been less powerful if I every time I called him and I just asked, "So what did you get up to yesterday?"

The difference between traditional goal setting and these strategies is subtle, but I have found that following this approach gives men more control over their sense of control, sense of progress and sense of success.

Ultimately, our aim is to help the men we care about to close the gap between who they are and who they want to be. There are only 2 ways that men can do that: make their goals more attainable; and make progress towards those goals. These 5 subtle changes do both and are the foundation of how I help my clients to feel more successful.

ENDNOTES

1 R239: Samaritans (2012). "Men and suicide: Why it's a social Issue." samaritans.org.
2 R158: Samaritans (2012). "Men, suicide and society: Why disadvantaged men in midlife die by suicide." samaritans.org.
3 R1456: Samaritans (2017). 'Dying from inequality: Socioeconomic disadvantage and suicidal behaviour.' Samaritans.org
4 R1366: O Remes et al. (2019). "Association between area deprivation and major depressive disorder in British men and women: a cohort study." BMJ Open.

5   R872: K Kosidou et al. (2011). "Socioeconomic status and risk of psychological distress and depression in the Stockholm Public Health Cohort: A population-based study." Journal of Affective Disorders.
6   R1540: A Preti (2007). "Suicide among animals: a review of evidence." Psychological Reports.
7   Brain serotonin is a complicated thing and very hard to measure. For the next few studies, by "brain serotonin levels" I am really talking about levels of 5-Hydroxyindoleacetic Acid (5HIAA) in the Cerebrospinal Fluid (CSF) of study participants. This is a metabolite of serotonin that can provide insights into serotonin activity in the brain.
8   R1265: J Hibbeln et al. (1998). "Essential fatty acids predict metabolites of serotonin and dopamine in cerebrospinal fluid among healthy control subjects, and early- and late-onset alcoholics." Biological Psychiatry.
9   R1260: P Nordström et al. (1994). "CSF 5-HIAA Predicts Suicide Risk After Attempted Suicide." Suicide and Life-Threatening Behaviour.
10 R1261: M Samuelsson et al. (2005). "CSF 5-HIAA, suicide intent and hopelessness in the prediction of early suicide in male high-risk suicide attempters." Acta Psychiatrica Scandinavica.
11 R1259: J J Mann & D Currier (2009). "Biological predictors of suicidal behaviour in mood disorders." Oxford Textbook of Suicidology and Suicide Prevention.
12 R103: M McGuire et al. (1984). "Behavioral and Physiological Correlates of Ostracism." Department of Psychiatry and Biobehavioral Sciences.
13 R103: M McGuire et al. (1984). "Behavioral and physiological correlates of ostracism." Department of Psychiatry and Biobehavioral Sciences.
14 Unfortunately, no one seems to have compared socioeconomic status with CSF 5HIAA levels in men, so we'll have to use other markers of serotonin activity for this chapter.
15 R677: K A Matthews et al. (2000). "Does Socioeconomic Status Relate to Central Serotonergic Responsivity in Healthy Adults?" Psychosomatic Medicine.
16 R1257: S Manuck et al. (2004). "The socio-economic status of communities predicts variation in brain serotonergic responsivity." Psychological Medicine.
17 R157: Samaritans (2020). "Out of sight, out of mind: Why less-well off, middle-aged men don't get the support they need." samaritans.org.
18 R702: G D Smith et al. (1990). "Magnitude and causes of socioeconomic differentials in mortality: further evidence from the Whitehall Study." Journal of Epidemiology & Community Health.
19 R703: M G Marmot et al. (1991). "Health inequalities among British civil servants: the Whitehall II study." The Lancet.
20 If it seems unlikely that serotonin could fluctuate based on how successful a man feels, later in the book we will explore how testosterone responds quickly when men believe they have won or lost a significant competition — illustrating how our hormones can react to perceptions of status or success.

21 R264: L Denneson et al. (2021). "Gender differences in recovery needs after a suicide attempt: a national qualitative study of US military veterans." Medical Care.
22 R1083: M Smith (2017). "Six in ten have failed to keep all their 2017 New Year's resolutions." YouGov.co.uk.
23 R377: Nina (2022). "How many people reach their goals? Goal statistics 2023." GoalsCalling.com.
24 R509: G Matthews (2015). "Research of Mean Goal Achievement." Dominican University

PART 3

LOOKING AFTER BODY & MIND

"The doctor of the future will give no medication but will interest his patients in the care of the human frame, diet and in the cause and prevention of disease."

– Thomas Edison

Looking After Body & Mind	
Signs of stress	-Feeling *down*, depressed -Low energy, poor sleep -Poor prostate health -High blood pressure -Poor heart health -Type 2 diabetes -Low libido, ED

Steve's story

Steve joined a coaching call with me because it was a condition from his wife, Andrea. He started by telling me that "It doesn't matter what you try to do with me, Ryan, because *even the doctors don't know what's wrong with me*. Everything is going wrong at the same time."

A year before we met, Steve had attended a health check where he was diagnosed with high blood pressure and advised to follow a low-fat diet to reduce his cholesterol levels. In particular, he was told to change his diet to avoid *saturated fat* – found in meat, cheese, and coconut oil. After 6 months on his low-fat diet, his cholesterol levels had reduced but his blood pressure had increased. He returned to the doctor's and was prescribed an additional blood pressure medication. Steve's doctor also found that Steve had high blood sugar and *HbA1c levels* and referred Steve to a diabetes specialist, who diagnosed Steve with *type 2 diabetes*.

Deflated, Steve gave up the diet. It seemed to him that there was no point following a diet if things kept going wrong. Andrea arranged for him to return to the doctor, who prescribed Steve SSRI antidepressants. Two weeks later – and for the first time – Steve started to think about ending his own life.

My first few phone calls with Steve focussed on getting him through a personal crisis. Then he decided to have some coaching calls to see whether it would help. As we spoke through The ALPHA Framework, he was particularly interested in the information about testosterone and physical health. Then it was time for our Future Call – the coaching exercise where Steve has to role-play a phone conversation after a successful and imaginary year.

Here is our conversation.

Steve's Future Call

Ryan: Ring-ring! Ring-ring! Ah, Steve. I wasn't expecting your call. How are you doing?

Steve: Hello, Ryan. Yes, I'm good, thank you. I've had quite an interesting year actually. The main thing that's happened is… I have realised that I am not broken.

[Steve shuffled in his chair for a moment and frowned at his keyboard. It was as if his own words were a surprise to him. His voice filled with emotion as he continued…]

Steve: When we first met last year, I *felt* broken. I kept getting hit with diagnosis after diagnosis. It was like my own health was a tomb that was falling in around me. I just felt so mortal all of a sudden. My strongest memory is of my doctor shaking his head and saying *"I'm not sure what's wrong with you"*. I was only forty-nine years old at the time. But things are so different now. It feels like a second chance at life. I feel young again.

[Steve carried on, telling me how positive he now felt about his health. Once I was confident that he was ready, I asked him 5 important coaching questions that I wanted him to answer.]

Ryan: Cast your mind back to when we had that very first Zoom call together one year ago… At the time, what was the main thing that was holding you back?

Steve: It was me. I had stopped looking after myself. Honestly, Ryan, if you had seen the nineteen-year-old me, you would have been impressed. I was so healthy and strong. I used to put in the effort. I looked after myself. Then, as I got older, I got complacent. I took my health for granted. I thought it was so unfair when my health started deteriorating, and yet I just sat there and let it happen. When we spoke last year, I wanted all the doctors and specialists and therapists to find my problem and fix it. But they couldn't, because the problem was me! I had to fix myself. I had to treat my health like it was something of value.

Ryan: What did you do to stop taking your health for granted and treat it like something of value?

Steve: I took small steps. For years I had been telling myself *"Next year I will join a gym"* and *"Next year I will make all my meals from scratch"*. But I never did. My energy was so low, I couldn't even start. Then, since our call last year, I have just been keeping it small and consistent – a short walk after dinner, taking an interest in what is actually in my food. It's just been the smallest changes that have made me feel so much better.

Ryan: Well done, Steve. You've had an amazing year, but I want to know: what has been the single best thing you've done all year?

Steve: I fit into my old suit and I watched my daughter graduate. She's the first one to do it in our family. And when she saw me back in my blue suit, she said, "I'm so proud of you, Dad." But she'll never know how proud I am of her. I had to start valuing my health, because I have to be around for her. I want to be here when she becomes a mum, and I want to be fit enough to play with my grandkids.

Ryan: If I had a time machine, and you could send a message back in time to be delivered to Steve at the end of his first coaching session one year ago, what would you say to him? What did he need to hear at the time?

Steve: I would say to him… *"Pull your finger out. You've got one life, one heart, one pair of legs. Don't let them waste away while you sit waiting for the next 'wonder drug' that's going to fix it all for you. Start small, but don't you dare give up on yourself. Because if you give up on your health, you're also giving up on your daughter and your wife. To look after them, you've got to look after yourself."*

Ryan: It's been an absolute honour seeing what you've achieved over the past year, Steve, but I want to know… Cast your mind back to that first coaching session we had a year ago. When you left the coaching call, what was the very first thing you did that got this amazing year off to a great start?

Steve: I sat down with Andrea and told her about our call. Then we planned some small changes that would make a big difference. All we did at first was have some walks after dinner and start to learn about the food we were putting into our bodies. But I felt better about myself. For the first time in years, I felt I had something I could do. I had some control over my health.

Ryan: Well done, Steve. You've had an amazing year and it's been my honour to watch you achieve so much. I know there were times where you made use of the expertise of others – friends, family, your doctor – but ultimately *YOU* made this happen. You realised what you really wanted and you went for it. And I want you to know that your daughter's proud of you, Andrea is proud of you, I'm proud of you, and you should be proud of yourself.

> Steve: Cheers, mate. I just needed that first kick up the backside.
>
> Ryan: Well, you did an awful lot with that kick, Steve. I have to go now, but it was great catching up.
>
> Steve: Goodbye, Ryan.
>
> Ryan: Goodbye, Steve.
> *BEEP*

The coaching exercise ended and Steve sat back in his chair with a hand on his chest, as if feeling his heart beat for the first time. "I have to say, I'm excited," he said. "When do we begin?"

The turning point for Steve was when he attended Hack Your Health — my workshop on boosting testosterone levels — as part of our work together. The day after attending, Steve's blood pressure reduced so much, he no longer needed one of his blood pressure medications (a *thiazide diuretic*). Ten days after the workshop, his morning testosterone levels had more than doubled from 4.4 to 9 nmol/L. Within 4 weeks, Steve's *HbA1c* (a marker for his average blood sugar levels over the past 3 months) had dropped from 59 to 45 mmol/mol. This meant that his type 2 diabetes was now in remission.

Over the following 8 weeks, his testosterone continued to rise while his waistline, heart health, and blood sugar all greatly improved. For Steve, focussing on his testosterone was key. It was easy to measure, responsive to his lifestyle changes and extremely motivating. It became the way that he kept score of his improving health. The reason this worked is because by improving his testosterone levels, he was also addressing the underlying cause of his other health problems: his metabolic health.

Metabolic health is how well your body stores, uses, and switches between different fuels for energy. It's an often-overlooked link between physical, mental, and hormonal health — so improving it can have more positive effects than you might expect.

Signs of poor metabolic health in men are: [1] [2] [3]

- Waist circumference greater than half his height (the waist measurement should be taken from 1" above the belly button – not his trouser size)
- Blood pressure over 140/90
- Fasting HDL-Cholesterol under 1 mmol/L
- Fasting triglycerides over 1.7 mmol/L
- Fasting blood glucose over 5.6 mmol/L

Because Steve had several of these signs, I knew some lifestyle changes would have a significant positive impact on his testosterone levels, and overall health.

Looking After Body & Mind is about the things men can do to improve and maintain their testosterone levels.

Looking After Body & Mind: The science

The decline of testosterone

The level of testosterone found in most men today is extremely low, compared to historical standards. Across the developed world, testosterone levels in men are declining every year; this means men today have much lower levels of testosterone than their grandfathers did at the same age.

Finnish Men in Their 60s

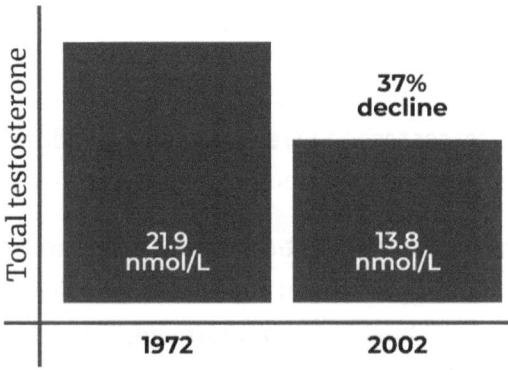

Adapted from R444: A Perheentupa et al. (2013) 'A cohort effect on serum testosterone levels in Finnish men.' *European Journal of Endocrinology.*

For example, a Finnish study found that in 1972, men in their 60s had a testosterone level of 21.9 nmol/L. But by 2002, men in their 60s in the same community had an average testosterone level of just 13.8 nmol/L. That's a decline of 37% in just 30 years! [4]

Multiple other European studies have found the same thing. A 2007 study compared 5,350 testosterone samples from the 1980s, 1990s, and early 2000s, finding "lower levels in the more recently born/studied men". [5,6]

This isn't only happening in Europe. An American study analysed 2,769 testosterone samples from 1,532 men living in Massachusetts and found that between 1987 and 2004, testosterone levels in men were consistently declining. The study concluded:

"These results indicate that recent years have seen a substantial, and as yet unrecognized, age-independent population-level decrease in testosterone in American men, potentially attributable to birth cohort differences or to health or environmental effects not captured in observed data." [7]

Essentially, this study found that:

1. testosterone levels are decreasing
2. they're not sure why, and
3. it's not even well known

This isn't only the case for older men; it's happening in younger men, too. Another study took data from the US National Health and Nutrition Examination Surveys (NHANES), focussing on young men (aged 15-39). They found that between the years 2000 and 2016, testosterone levels in young men declined from an average of 21 nmol/L to 15.6. That's a 26% decline in 16 years. [8]

And in 2014, a study published in *PLOS One* stated that testosterone peaks in 19-year-olds **at 15.4 nmol/L**. That means the 19-year-olds in this study had lower levels of testosterone than their great-grandads probably had when they were 60 years old! [9]

In case you didn't read part 1, or you need a recap, the answer to the question *"What is a healthy level of testosterone?"* depends on who you ask.

Many labs and healthcare providers today will advise men that testosterone levels as low as 12 nmol/L - or even 6.8 - are normal. Some will even use words like "optimal" which I find very misleading.

I think that men over 18 should at least have testosterone levels as high as 60-year-old men used to have: and that's 20 nmol/L. Below that may have indeed become normal, but normal isn't the same as good.

So why are testosterone levels declining in men? And what can we do about it?

Nowadays you will hear many theories ranging from the widespread use of the contraceptive pill increasing oestrogen in the water to microplastics in our bodies blocking production of testosterone in men. I'm not suggesting that these things don't have an impact, but there is something more obvious – and more useful – for us to focus on.

The factor I am talking about explains why low testosterone is linked to the biggest killers of men. I believe it explains why testosterone levels tend to decline as men age *and* why they are decreasing every year in men the same age. By addressing this single factor, men can beat the downwards trends and quickly, naturally, and very significantly increase their testosterone levels.

That factor is *insulin resistance*.

Why low testosterone is so dangerous for men

Insulin resistance impacts different organs in different ways. But wherever it occurs, it causes problems: in the **muscles** it can cause blood sugar to rise and the pancreas to struggle, leading to a condition called *type 2 diabetes*. [10]

Insulin resistance also causes your **kidneys** to store salts, which can lead to a condition called "*salt sensitive hypertension*", where salt in your food raises your blood pressure, meaning you have to monitor your salt intake. [11][12]

In the **liver**, insulin resistance leads to the build-up of fat. If the insulin resistance was caused by alcohol, it's called "*alcoholic fatty liver disease*". When it occurs in children and people who don't drink, it's called "*non-alcoholic fatty liver disease*". [13] The combination of these fats being released by the liver, plus high blood pressure, may speed up the development of heart disease and the risk of heart failure. [14]

Emerging evidence is starting to suggest that insulin resistance in the **brain** is linked to depression, bipolar disorder, epilepsy, schizophrenia, and Alzheimer's. [15][16][17][18]

In men, insulin resistance has been linked to biological changes that can contribute to an enlarged prostate and erectile dysfunction (ED). In women, Insulin resistance is also associated with polycystic ovary syndrome (PCOS) – symptoms include irregular periods, infertility, and higher testosterone levels (yes, the opposite to men). [19][20][21]

Many cancers are associated with insulin resistance, including pancreatic cancer, which has the lowest survival rate of any cancer. [22]

Insulin resistance has also been linked to less serious but often overlooked symptoms—such as difficulty concentrating, poor mental stamina, and feeling sleepy or drowsy during the day (especially after a meal containing carbohydrates). [23]

In many of these mental and physical health issues, reducing insulin resistance can reduce the symptoms or even reverse the condition. And if you don't have these conditions, reducing insulin resistance will significantly reduce your risk of developing them in the first place.

All this is especially relevant to my mission, because the conditions mentioned in this chapter (from depression to heart disease, type 2 diabetes to high blood pressure, schizophrenia to enlarged prostate) are all associated with increased risk of suicide. And that is probably because insulin resistance itself is associated with suicide. [24][25][26][27][28]

What's all this got to do with testosterone? Well, I've given examples of how insulin resistance shows up and affects different organs in the body, and most of a man's testosterone is made in his testicles. When the testosterone-making cells in the testicle become insulin resistant, they make less testosterone. These cells appear to be so sensitive, that low testosterone may be the earliest warning sign of insulin resistance in men. [29][30][31][32]

At the start of this book, I showed that low testosterone is linked to the biggest killers of men — suicide, heart disease, cancer, and Alzheimer's. Here's why this matters:

- Insulin resistance is a key factor behind many of these serious health problems.
- Low testosterone is often an early warning sign that insulin resistance is developing.
- Recognising that low testosterone is a sign of insulin resistance in men could lead to better prevention and save lives.

Despite the known link between low testosterone and insulin resistance, many of the brilliant people I know who work in healthcare, mental health or suicide prevention haven't been taught about this relationship.

In the UK's National Confidential Inquiry into Suicide and Safety in Mental Health, it was found:

"More than half (52%) of men who died [from suicide] had a physical health condition, most commonly circulatory system diseases, such as hypertension. We ask services to be aware of the importance of physical ill-health as a factor in suicide risk. We suggest that help-seeking for physical health problems may be an opportunity for prevention." [33]

I'm pleased that the research is making people aware of the link between poor physical health and suicide. But just knowing the link exists isn't enough: we have to start helping men address the underlying factor. Everything I've told you is publicly available information in respected medical journals, but not part of standard training for many healthcare, diet, or mental health professionals.

So, now you know that insulin resistance is a big problem for our physical and mental health. But how do we reduce insulin resistance? To answer that, we need to explore what causes it in the first place.

How low-carb impacts testosterone in men

To understand insulin resistance, we first have to understand insulin.

Your body is made out of trillions of cells. These cells need energy, otherwise they will die. They get this energy from the food you eat, specifically from fat (which is broken down into fatty acids, and an energy source known as "*ketones*") and carbohydrates (sugar and starch, both broken down into an energy source called "*glucose*").

From now on, I'll refer to fat, fatty acids and ketones as simply "fat" and sugar, starch, and glucose as simply "sugar".

Most of the cells in your body can switch between burning fat and burning sugar, depending on what's available. However, current dietary guidelines in the UK and US encourage us to get the majority of our energy from carbohydrates and to limit fat intake.

Foods high in carbohydrates — which range from sweets, chocolate, and sugary drinks to pasta, rice, and porridge — are broken down into sugar, which enters your bloodstream. A high blood sugar level is harmful, and so your body carefully regulates it. To give some perspective: when your blood sugar is at a healthy level (around 5 mmol/L), there is only about 4.5g sugar circulating in your entire bloodstream — roughly a teaspoon. For context, a medium-sized banana contains about 6× that amount of sugar.

As a result, when you eat carbohydrates, your body must act quickly to keep your blood sugar in check: that's where insulin comes in. Insulin is a hormone produced and then released by your pancreas to block fat burning and order cells to take in the sugar from your bloodstream. Some of that sugar is used for immediate energy, but if the cells receive more than they can use, the rest is stored. Your body has very limited sugar (glycogen) stores, so once those are full, excess sugar is converted into fat. This new fat may circulate in the blood (called "*triglycerides*"), be stored under the skin ("*subcutaneous fat*"), or accumulate around internal organs ("*visceral fat*"). In this way, high-carbohydrate diets can cause your body to store more and more fat. [34]

Food guidelines in the UK suggest we should "Base meals on potatoes, bread, rice, pasta or other starchy carbohydrates" and choose lower-fat options. This means that many of us are eating carbohydrates with every meal. A 150g serving of potato or rice has been found to increase blood sugar levels as much as 9–10 teaspoons of pure white sugar. The result is that our pancreas is working to remove large amounts of sugar from our blood several times a day. [35] [36] [37]

Your body is a delicate balancing act and when you have too much of something, your cells can start to become less sensitive to it.

A good example of this is alcohol. Have you ever noticed that people who drink alcohol regularly get drunk slower? While those of us who don't drink alcohol get drunk very quickly? When your cells become less sensitive to alcohol, we call it alcohol *tolerance*. In a similar way, when your cells are exposed to high levels of insulin over a long period, they become less sensitive to it. Rather than call this insulin tolerance, it's called insulin resistance. [38] [39]

While there are many factors thought to cause insulin resistance – from sleep deprivation to chronic stress and exposure to radiation – one of the most common factors is simply long-term high levels of insulin.

Once cells become resistant to insulin, they take up less sugar from the blood. In response, the pancreas produces more insulin to try to keep blood sugar at a healthy level. These higher insulin levels encourage the body to store more fat and make it harder to burn fat for energy, while also causing more insulin resistance. Over time, this cycle can strain the pancreas and it can't produce enough insulin to counter the high blood sugar. This is what had happened to Steve, leaving him with type 2 diabetes, high blood pressure and low testosterone.

Even in men who do not have symptoms of insulin resistance, it appears large amounts of carbohydrates can temporarily reduce testosterone. In one experiment published in *Clinical Endocrinology* in 2012, 74 men were given 75g of glucose (the form of sugar that our bodies get from bread, pasta, rice, and porridge). Testosterone levels dropped by 25% for at least 2 hours

– we don't know whether they returned to normal that day. This significant reduction was not only in men with insulin resistance and type 2 diabetes, but also in healthy men without insulin resistance. For context, 2 medium-sized bottles of Lucozade Original contain more than 75g of glucose. [40] [41]

While this all may sound concerning, there is good news: studies show that insulin resistance can often be improved – and in some cases reversed, just like Steve did. One effective strategy is to encourage the body to shift back into fat-burning mode, also known as *ketosis*. [42]

To achieve ketosis, you can change **when** you eat (fasting) or can change **what** you eat (a ketogenic diet).

The most common form of fasting is probably *intermittent fasting* – where you eat all your meals for the day in an 8 hour window, leaving time for insulin levels to return to normal. If you are used to eating a low-carbohydrate diet, intermittent fasting is often comfortable. However, if you are used to eating carbohydrates with every meal, even intermittent fasting can be challenging as fluctuating blood sugar levels can leave you feeling hungry throughout the day.

Even without fasting, you can still reduce your natural insulin levels simply by eating less carbohydrates. Eating less than 130g of carbohydrates per day is often referred to as 'low-carb'. The level at which ketosis kicks in varies in everyone, but it's generally between 30 and 50g of carbohydrates per day. This means not all low-carb diets are ketogenic. [43]

Ketogenic diets have long been used as a way to manage epilepsy, reverse type 2 diabetes, and to lose weight. But more recently they are being recommended by healthcare professionals to improve outcomes of other conditions associated with insulin resistance, like bipolar disorder, schizoaffective disorder, major depressive disorder, PCOS, and some forms of cancer. [44] [45] [46] [47] [48] [49] [50] [51]

I first became aware of ketogenic diets when I was learning what to eat to boost my testosterone. Several studies came out in 2020 exploring what happens when men with low testosterone follow a ketogenic diet combined with intermittent fasting.

In 1 study, 20 men took their average testosterone levels from 6.5 nmol/L to about 13 nmol/L, in 12 weeks. Yes, you read that correctly. Their testosterone *doubled* in 12 weeks. The increase in testosterone was accompanied by significant improvements in insulin and insulin resistance. [52]

In another study, 34 obese men took their average testosterone levels from 13.2 nmol/L to 17.2 nmol/L in 12 weeks – from low to around average. This increase in testosterone was accompanied by a 90% increase in vitamin D, 75% reduction in insulin resistance, 48% reduction in their blood triglycerides, and significant improvements in blood sugar, insulin, weight, BMI, waist circumference, PSA, and liver health. [53]

A third study took 25 college-aged men and divided them into 2 groups. One group followed a ketogenic diet for 10 weeks. Their testosterone levels increased from 19.7 nmol/L to 23.8 nmol/L. The other group followed their normal carbohydrate-based diet and experienced a slight reduction in their testosterone levels. The study concluded:

"The ketogenic diet can be used in combination with resistance training to cause favorable changes in body composition, performance, and hormonal profiles in resistance-trained men." [54]

These are all small studies, but they all point in the same direction: cutting down the amount of carbohydrates that men eat is an easy, effective, and natural way to increase testosterone levels. In 2023, a review published in *Endocrine* pulled together the findings from 7 studies that included 230 participants, and also found that ketogenic diets significantly and consistently improved testosterone levels in men. [55]

After learning this, I decided to try the same thing in my own body and followed a ketogenic (low-carbohydrate, high-fat) diet for 12 weeks. I had no calorie limit, just a limit on carbohydrates.

I could see straight away that it was going to be quite a big change. Almost everything that came out of a packet was full of carbohydrates. It was no longer going to be possible to eat processed foods or anything sold by "convenience" stores. In practice, a low-carbohydrate diet meant that I had to eat lots of natural "whole" foods.

For the first few days, I felt a bit sluggish because my body wasn't used to burning fat. But by day 4, I felt excellent. My body had kicked into fat-burning mode. I no longer felt painfully hungry when I woke up, no longer felt snackish between meals and I no longer felt tired after lunch.

I went from needing 3 meals a day (plus snacks) just to function, to feeling satisfied with just 2 meals and no snacks. After the first 12 weeks my morning testosterone levels increased slightly from 20.4 nmol/L to 23.3 nmol/L. A nice little increase, but not as impressive as the studies I mentioned earlier – probably because I was already in good metabolic health.

But I felt so good, that I decided to carry on with the diet indefinitely. After 8 months of ketosis, my morning testosterone levels had risen to 29.7 nmol/L. At the time, I had never met a man with testosterone levels that high! And not only had my testosterone levels improved, but also my blood sugar, heart health, and energy levels greatly improved. [56]

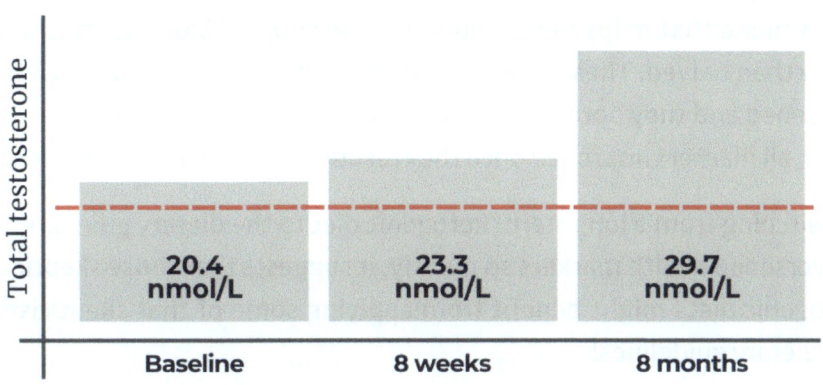

R1455: R Parke (2025). "Hack Your Health." TheMensCoach.co.uk.
Dotted line represents median average for healthy males aged 18-39.

This is why I don't use phrases like "male menopause" or "andropause" when it comes to low testosterone levels in men. Menopause in women is an inevitable part of ageing, and can't be reversed. But in men, low testosterone is not an ageing problem; it is a lifestyle problem. And it can be addressed very quickly if you know how.

The only difficulty I had when I started a low-carb diet was with salt. When you follow a low-carbohydrate diet, your body stores less salt and water. This means you might have to start adding salt to your diet, especially if you are very active. Low salt levels can lead to muscle cramps, light-headedness, or – in extreme cases – death. Because I was exercising very regularly, I found I needed to start drinking fasting salts in water to avoid getting muscle cramps. I include the link to the salts I used on TheMensCoach.co.uk/resources. [57]

Low-carb diets are often seen as a short-term (but unsustainable) option, with some people concerned about the long term health implications. But one recent study in particular challenges that idea. Dr Isabella Cooper and her team studied 10 healthy women who had been in ketosis for years. For 21 days, these women stopped following their ketogenic diet and instead ate according to the UK's dietary guidelines, which recommends carbohydrates with every meal. [58]

During those 21 days, insulin levels increased, blood sugar rose, and the women gained weight. Insulin resistance more than doubled and GLP-1 (a hormone that helps reduce appetite and support blood sugar control) more than halved. These changes suggest the women's metabolic health worsened and they potentially became more prone to hunger. Encouragingly, all markers improved once they resumed their usual ketogenic diet.

If switching from a long-term ketogenic diet to the dietary guidelines led to worsened health markers so quickly, it suggests that those skeptical of ketogenic diets might benefit from applying some of that skepticism to the dietary guidelines!

Here are the key points from this section so far:

- In men, low testosterone is an early sign of a bigger problem: insulin resistance.
- Insulin resistance is associated with depression, suicide, heart disease, many cancers, and Alzheimer's (the biggest killers of men).
- You can reduce insulin resistance by getting into fat-burning mode (ketosis), either through a ketogenic diet or through fasting.

- Fat-burning mode can significantly increase testosterone levels in men.
- If you have a medical condition, mental health condition, or take medication, speak to your healthcare provider before you change your diet as ketosis can quickly change how much medication or salt you need.

But hold on a minute, surely you have to be careful not to eat too much fat, because it's bad for your health?

I thought that too, until I looked for evidence of it.

How low-fat and low cholesterol impact life expectancy

There is some disagreement between experts as to whether low-fat or low-carb diets are best for us. Before I learned about hormonal health, I used to believe that a low-fat diet (especially, being low in *saturated* fat) is good for our health. After all, that's what I had always been told growing up. But when I started to look for evidence to support this belief, I kept finding information that low-fat is not necessarily good for us.

Studies like this one kept coming up:

The Prospective Urban Rural Epidemiology (PURE) study followed 135,355 people in 18 countries. Participants reported what they ate, and the study followed up for over 7 years to see who died, had a heart attack, heart disease, or stroke throughout the study. [59]

Here's what the study found:

- Those who ate the highest amounts of fat were **21% less likely to die** during the study period than those eating the lowest amounts.
- Those who ate the highest amounts of carbohydrate were **28% more likely to die** during the study period than those eating the lowest amounts.
- Neither total fat nor types of fat were associated with heart disease.
- Those who ate the highest amount of **saturated fat** were **14% less likely to die** during the study period than those who ate the lowest amounts.

- Those who ate the highest amount of **saturated fat** were **21% less likely to have a stroke** than those who ate the least.

In essence, over 1 million years of data (135,355 people multiplied by 7.4 years) could be summarised in 2 sentences: *The more fat you eat, the longer you live. The more carbohydrates you eat, the shorter you live.*

The study was published in world-respected scientific journal *The Lancet* with the very strong wording: *"Global dietary guidelines should be reconsidered in light of these findings."*

The "guidelines" the article is referring to are the current dietary guidelines to avoid food like butter, full fat dairy, and red meat, because they contain saturated fat.

Of course, this is only one study, and (like every study) it has its limitations. But the findings of the PURE study are not unique. For example, a 2010 article published in *The American Journal of Clinical Nutrition* reviewed 21 studies on saturated fat, including a total of 347,747 people. Like the PURE study, the analysis found that **more saturated fat** was associated with **lower risk of stroke.**

It concluded that the analysis had *"showed that there is no significant evidence for concluding that dietary saturated fat is associated with an increased risk of [heart disease or stroke]."* [60]

Another 2010 study of 53,644 Danish men and women found that **each 5% reduction in saturated fat was associated with a 33% increase in heart attacks** if that saturated fat was replaced by **carbohydrates with a high glycemic index** — foods that cause fast spikes in blood sugar, typically including white bread, many breakfast cereals, white rice, and some types of potatoes. And a study of 1,036 adults found that eating saturated fat was associated with **better heart health,** unless it was combined with a high-carbohydrate diet. [61] [62]

In 2020, the *Journal of the American College of Cardiology* published a comprehensive and up-to-date overview on the matter:

"The recommendation to limit dietary [saturated fat] intake has persisted despite mounting evidence to the contrary. Most recent meta-analyses of

randomized trials and observational studies found no beneficial effects of reducing [saturated fat] intake on cardiovascular disease (CVD) and total mortality, and instead found protective effects against stroke. [...] It is also apparent that the health effects of foods cannot be predicted by their content in any nutrient group without considering the overall macronutrient distribution. Whole-fat dairy, unprocessed meat, and dark chocolate are [saturated fat]-rich foods with a complex matrix that are not associated with increased risk of CVD. The totality of available evidence does not support further limiting the intake of such foods." [63]

Why does this matter? Because treating natural sources of saturated fat as unhealthy drives people toward highly processed alternatives — margarines, refined seed oils, low-fat snacks, and sugary cereals — swapping real, nutrient-rich foods for artificial substitutes.

So saturated fat doesn't seem to be dangerous, and may reduce our risk of stroke. In contrast, studies show that eating less fat can:

- reduce HDL-cholesterol (often known as "good cholesterol"),
- increase triglycerides (fat stores in the blood), and
- reduce testosterone levels in men.

These are all things associated with **worse heart health**. [64] [65] [66] [67] [68]

So if eating less fat can have these negative effects, why then was Steve advised to follow a low-fat diet? Firstly, to lose weight. But it's worth knowing that an analysis of 71 weight-loss trials which compared *low-fat* with *low-carb* diets found that low-carb diets were more effective in 62 trials, and significantly more effective in 39. Many of the trials also found that low-carb diets led to greater improvements in blood sugar, HDL ("good") cholesterol and triglycerides, compared to the low-fat diets. Many of these trials didn't even include ketogenic diets; they were simply keeping carbohydrates below 130g per day. Low-fat diets were more effective in 7 studies, **significantly more effective in none** - and in 1 trial, the low-fat group actually gained weight. So it seems that a low-carb diet could have been better for Steve in the first place. [69]

Secondly, Steve had been told that his cholesterol was creeping up, and that eating less fat could bring it down. He had been told that people with lower cholesterol are less likely to die from heart disease, which is a very compelling reason to make changes!

But does that mean that people with low cholesterol actually live longer overall?

To answer that, we need to look at cholesterol in some detail...

Cholesterol is a vital building block that your cells are made out of. Your body needs cholesterol to make new cells, repair old cells, and make important hormones (like testosterone and oestrogen). Cholesterol is so important that almost all the cells in your body can make their own cholesterol if there isn't enough of it in your blood. [70][71]

In your blood, cholesterol travels inside particles called lipoproteins ('lipo' means fat, so a 'lipoprotein' is made from fat and protein). You can think of different lipoproteins as different bus routes, each carrying cholesterol to various parts of your body for different jobs:

- HDL ('high-density lipoprotein') cholesterol is often called "good" cholesterol because it's linked to better heart health.
- LDL ('low-density lipoprotein') cholesterol is often called "bad" cholesterol, but this is an oversimplification because there are several types of LDL. They're not all bad - and some are good - but most tests don't differentiate them. [72]
- Triglycerides are fats stored in your blood to be used for energy. They're not cholesterol, but they're often measured at the same time.

No single measurement tells the whole story of heart health, but some ratios can give useful insights into heart risk and metabolic health. Probably the most useful ratios are the triglyceride to HDL cholesterol (TG:HDL) ratio, and the total cholesterol to HDL cholesterol (TC:HDL) ratio. [73]

'Total' cholesterol is the number you get when you add up all the cholesterol carried by the different lipoproteins (bus routes). That single number hides the important details that really matter for understanding heart health.

Despite this, most cholesterol conversations focus on *total* cholesterol. In the UK, the NHS advises that **a healthy level of total cholesterol is "below 5 mmol/L"**. [74]

But recent evidence seriously challenges this guidance - especially for men over the age of 35.

In 2019, a Korean study was published in *Scientific Reports* that analysed total cholesterol levels and "all-cause mortality" (death from any cause, not just heart disease). The study took total cholesterol measured during routine health check-ups between 2001 and 2004, then checked which of those people died before 2013 – an average follow-up of 10.5 years.

By comparing total cholesterol levels with mortality over the next decade, the study aimed to understand how well total cholesterol levels could predict life expectancy.

How many people were included in the study?

12,815,006 people.

Yes, 12.8 million people. This is an absolutely enormous study. The graph below shows the full results, split by sex. I've also added men aged 45-54 as a separate line: [75]

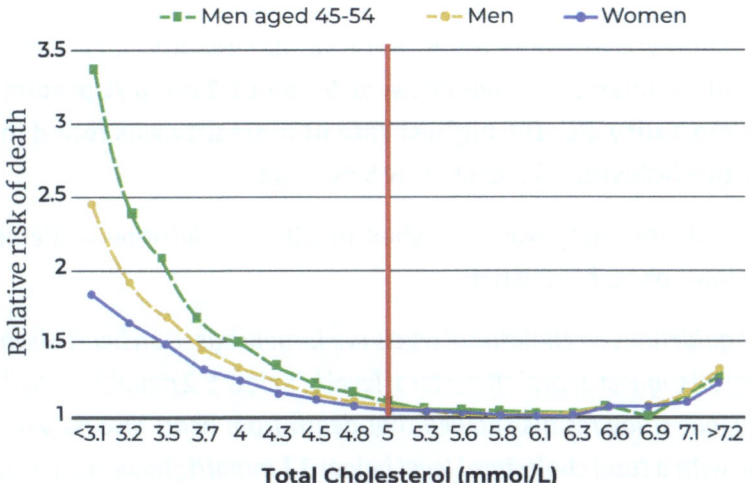

Adapted from R652: S-W Yi (2019). 'Total cholesterol and all-cause mortality by sex and age: a prospective cohort study among 12.8 million adults.' *Scientific Reports*. Ryan has added a vertical line at 5 mmol/L because UK guidelines recommend that a total cholesterol of below 5 mmol/L is 'healthy'.

The study found that in men over the age of 35:

- Mortality was **lowest** in those with a total cholesterol of 5.4 to 6.4 mmol/L.
- Mortality was **highest** in those with the lowest total cholesterol.

In men aged 45-54 (Steve's age group), low total cholesterol was associated with a very high rate of mortality. Those with the lowest total cholesterol levels were 3.5× more likely to die in the following 10 years, compared to those who had 'borderline high' cholesterol. [76]

Because this article uses a different measurement for cholesterol, and a lot of scientific names for diseases, I've paraphrased their findings below:

The current cholesterol guidelines are heavily based on heart disease risk and recommend a cholesterol level of <5.2 mmol/L as desirable. A cholesterol level below 5.2 mmol/L, however, may not be necessarily a sign of good health when other diseases are considered.

This enormous study challenges the common belief that "*lower is better*" when it comes to total cholesterol. And it even questions whether "below 5 mmol/L" is healthy at all for men over 35 or women over 45. But it's still only 1 study. Next let's look at a study that uses US data…

Analysis of 25,429 US adults in the National Health and Nutrition Examination Survey (NHANES) found very similar results. Like the Korean study, total cholesterol levels between 5.1 and 7.2 mmol/L **predicted the lowest mortality**. But the **highest rate of mortality was found in those with total cholesterol levels below 5 mmol/L.** [77]

Analysis of the study was published in 2021 in *Nutrition & Metabolism*, which I have paraphrased here:

Current guidelines on cholesterol levels are largely based on heart disease risk, and they all suggest a total cholesterol level of below 5.2 mmol/L is ideal. Interestingly, our study results showed that death from heart disease was lowest in those with a total cholesterol level below 3.1 mmol/L; however, a total cholesterol level of below 5.2 mmol/L was strongly linked to a higher risk of death from all causes, as well as cancer.

I know it looks like I have accidentally repeated the findings from the Korean study, but I haven't – this US data simply found the same thing. Unlike the Korean study, this study of American data recorded certain causes of death – specifically heart disease or cancer. I've used the University of Cambridge's RealRisk tool to show what the figures actually mean in real numbers:

Deaths Per 100 People* over the following 15 years						
Total Cholesterol at baseline	<3.1 mmol/L	3.1 - 4.1 mmol/L	4.1 - 5.1 mmol/L	5.1 - 6.2 mmol/L	6.2 - 7.2 mmol/L	>7.2 mmol/L
Heart disease	1	1	1	1	1	2
Cancer	4	2	2	1	1	2
Any cause	14	10	7	7	6	8

*The participants **had not been diagnosed with heart disease or cancer** at the beginning of the study.

Adapted from R1293: G He et al. (2021). "A nonlinear association of total cholesterol with all-cause and cause-specific mortality." *Nutrition & Metabolism*. Relative risks were converted to absolute risk per 100 people using the RealRisk tool (realrisk.wintoncentre.uk), the baseline risk from the reference range (160–199 mg/dL) and the hazard ratios (HRs) from Model III on "Table 2 Multivariate Cox regression analysis of total cholesterol levels with cause-specific mortality". Ryan then converted the mg/dL units into mmol/L and rounded the results to the nearest whole person.

When you look at death from all-causes (rather than focussing only on heart disease), lower total cholesterol is not necessarily better. The studies and organisations that are advising us to keep total cholesterol below 5 mmol/L are focussing only on heart disease and disregarding overall health. I think this is very important to understand, because almost 9 out of 10 UK men will be **killed by something other than heart disease**. [78]

I was so intrigued by the Korean study's finding that middle-aged men with low cholesterol had the highest mortality that I began exploring other research on cholesterol in this age group.

In a 12-year study of 350,977 middle-aged men, it was found that:

"A [total] cholesterol level less than 4.14 mmol/L was also associated with a significantly increased risk of death from cancer of the liver and pancreas;

digestive diseases, particularly hepatic cirrhosis; **suicide;** *and alcohol dependence syndrome. In addition, [the lower the cholesterol level, the higher the rate of] cancers of the lung, lymphatic, and hematopoietic systems, and chronic obstructive pulmonary disease."* (I made the word suicide bold for my own emphasis) [79]

Yes, you read that correctly: suicide.

In 1992, a study published in *The British Medical Journal* found that low total cholesterol was associated with a 4.2× higher risk of suicide in men. In 2001, a study published in *Epidemiology* found that those with a low total cholesterol level may be 6× more likely to die from suicide. There have been other studies between these 2, but you get the idea. Still, in 2025, men are often advised that below 5 mmol/L is a "healthy" level of total cholesterol for everyone. [80] [81]

It seems to me that low total cholesterol protects you from heart disease in the same way that being hit by a bus protects you from heart disease: you are just less likely to live long enough to develop heart disease.

That might sound like a flippant comment, but it highlights a real problem: much health advice and research focuses on a single outcome—like heart disease—without considering overall health. When advice is based on such a narrow view, it can be misleading, even when it comes from trusted organisations.

Enough about cholesterol studies and what I think - what did Steve decide to do?

After learning about insulin, insulin resistance, and cholesterol, Steve could understand why his low-fat diet had led to reduced total cholesterol, high blood pressure and a new diagnosis of type 2 diabetes. Eating less fat and more carbohydrates had worsened his metabolic health!

The day after attending Hack Your Health, Steve swapped his low-fat breakfast of overnight oats, raisins, and a banana for a low-carb, high-fat breakfast of salmon, avocado, and cream cheese. Normally, his blood pressure would rise after eating and by 11 a.m. he'd need his medication – a thiazide diuretic. But after this breakfast, his blood pressure stayed in the normal range. He called his doctor, who advised him not to take the medication that day, since his blood pressure was already healthy.

One meal in and already noticing a difference, Steve began tracking his blood pressure readings more closely. He has since monitored his blood pressure daily, and - at the point of writing this - has not needed that medication again.

Steve's doctor didn't understand why Steve was doing a low-carb diet (eating that much fat seemed *dangerous* to him), but he was pleased to see Steve's health improve. Steve shared some articles with him to answer his doctor's questions about low-carb diets and then they safely tapered Steve's medications together.

Just by addressing his insulin resistance through his diet, Steve also addressed his high blood pressure, his type 2 diabetes, and his low testosterone levels. After 3 weeks, he felt so much better he started working with his doctor to safely taper his antidepressants.

Important: If you – or someone you know – takes medication and wants to improve their health using a ketogenic diet or fasting, but your doctor or dietitian isn't familiar with these approaches, there are resources available to help.

The University of Manitoba and the *British Journal of General Practice* have both published helpful guides for healthcare professionals on how to safely reduce and discontinue medications when a patient starts and follows a low-carb diet. These guides explain the science behind ketogenic diets and fasting in a way that helps doctors understand why your health can quickly improve — and how to adjust medications accordingly.

You can find these resources on the "Tools for Healthcare Practitioners" section of my Resources page: TheMensCoach.co.uk/resources

I'll say it again: it's essential to work with your healthcare provider if you take medication. A ketogenic diet can address the root cause of many chronic issues, but, if you take medication, that also means you could quickly become over-medicated, which can be dangerous.

Steve's story is a brilliant example: after just one lifestyle change, he had to stop one of his blood pressure medications — with the proper medical supervision.

About a month later, Steve was invited by his local NHS Trust to a training session to help him manage his diabetes. The trainers were surprised when he told them he was already in remission.

During the training, he was told that a **total cholesterol level below 5 mmol/L is good** — but that 3.1 mmol/L is considered ideal, because people with total cholesterol that low have the lowest risk of dying from heart disease.

Fortunately, by that point, Steve had learned enough to understand the nuance behind that claim. When he asked how a total cholesterol level of below 5 mmol/L affects life expectancy in men, the trainer paused — and then honestly admitted, "*I don't know.*"

We live in a world where saturated fat, cholesterol, and testosterone are often demonised. Issues relating to insulin resistance are rising while testosterone in men is falling. Much of today's health advice remains a one-size-fits-all approach, lacking the nuance that can make all the difference — not only to male hormonal, mental, and physical health, but to many different groups and individuals.

I'm confident the official guidelines will one day catch up, but in the meantime...

Are we paying the price?

Testosterone: The male "capability" hormone

So far, I hope to have made the argument that testosterone is a hormone that responds to lifestyle and can offer key insights into a man's physical and mental health. But there is another very important factor influencing testosterone levels: competition. This is crucial to understand, because the dynamics of competition can shift testosterone within minutes — creating either a powerful way to help him feel better, or a significant risk to his health.

To explain this, the best place to start is with monkeys.

Just like men, male monkeys have a baseline level of testosterone that's impacted by their overall health and social status. But this can change very quickly...

Let's say 2 monkeys spot 1 delicious meal, only big enough for 1 of them to eat. Now that there is a challenge, the testosterone level in both monkeys will begin to increase to around 4× the baseline. [82]

What happens next depends on the outcome. Let's say 1 monkey is a little bit more street smart than the other; he flashes his sharp monkey teeth, and the other monkey thinks, "Screw that, it's not worth it," and runs away. Testosterone levels in the monkey who clearly won the challenge increase by a staggering further 20%. His testosterone is now many times higher than before the competition, so he is feeling particularly good about himself.

But for the monkey who lost the challenge, his testosterone levels will come crashing down by around 90% – meaning they are now significantly lower than the baseline levels of testosterone before the competition.

Which made me wonder, if this is how challenge impacts testosterone in monkeys, what does it do in men?

Several studies suggest similar results. A small experiment involving 6 male tennis players, and a study involving a group of male chess players have found that testosterone significantly fluctuates during competition – with winning driving testosterone up and losing driving it down. [83] [84]

So competing and winning seems to increase testosterone in men, but is that due to the fact victory was *earned* or *perceived*? In 2018, a study published in *Human Nature* tried to answer that. The study paired up 42 healthy male rowers in a direct indoor rowing competition with a similarly skilled opponent. One week before the contest, these rowers completed a health assessment – including testosterone measurements. On the day of the competition, the rowers could not see their opponent's performance during the race. At the end of the race, rather than announcing the "true" winner, victory was randomly assigned to one of the competitors. [85]

The study found that testosterone significantly increased in those who believed they won, and decreased in those who believed they lost. The experiment also collected other interesting results. Those who believed they won also had an increase in their self-confidence, their self-assessed value as a mate, and were found to be more inclined to approach a woman they found attractive for a potential date (compared to their own questionnaire answers from the week before). Four of the rowers – two "winners" and two "losers" – suspected that the results had been manipulated, and their results were excluded from the analysis.

It appears that, just like in the monkeys, testosterone levels in men increase when they are challenged and when they believe they have won, but decrease when they believe they have lost. Which leads me on to my favourite study on testosterone of all…

In 1994, the FIFA World Cup final was Brazil versus Italy. Researchers travelled to bars where Brazilian and Italian male fans were watching the game. These men were not playing, they weren't even playing chess, they were just watching a very meaningful game (in football terms). [86][87]

Baseline levels of testosterone were taken from these men 25 to 15 minutes before the game began and then 15 to 25 minutes after the winners were announced. After the game, testosterone levels in Brazilian male fans had increased by more than 25%. During the same time period, testosterone levels in Italian male fans decreased by more than 25%. Can you guess who won?

Male Fans Watching 1994 World Cup

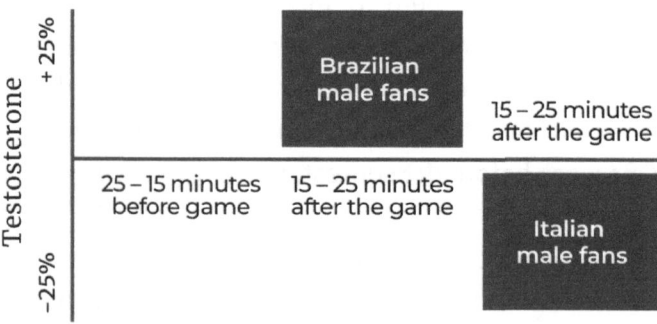

Adapted from R253: C Suplee (1995). 'Score One for the Hormone Team '*Washington Post*'.

You guessed it: Brazil.

This suggests that – just from watching a sports team they identify with – men go on the same hormonal and emotional roller coaster as they would go through if they were actually taking part themselves. (This isn't an excuse for bad behaviour, by the way, only an attempt to explain part of what might make up the "post-match blues" in men who see their team lose.)

And given that Brazil won when Italy missed a penalty in the final second of gameplay, this means that the hormones only had around 15 minutes to react, so we know that these fluctuations happen within minutes, not hours.

Knowing what you know now about how low testosterone predicts heart attack risk in men, what do you think happens to rates of heart attacks on days when sports teams lose? You probably guessed it…

Many studies have found that on days where their sports teams lose, fatal heart attacks and strokes in male fans increase by between 29% and 51%. [88] [89]

Over the years, I have heard many men's health organisations explain this phenomenon as being the result of "stress". But if you are familiar with the studies, you can see this isn't correct. Because when men watch a stressful game that their team wins, there is no increase in heart attacks. The risk is associated with the meaningful loss, not the stress. [90]

And the same research suggests that there is no increased risk of heart attack in female fans, regardless of the result. [91]

This is a real and worrying issue.

Thankfully, there is a solution. I've worked with many men who have overcome the post-loss blues simply by watching old videos of their team's previous triumphant performance. Sometimes the videos are very old, but that doesn't seem to make them less effective.

I think that these sports studies can act as a beautiful metaphor for how external factors – challenge, meaningful wins, and meaningful losses

— impact the hormonal health and the mental health of the men we care about.

Understanding the role of competition — and how winning or losing affects testosterone — is a vital part of Looking After Body & Mind. Hormones in men react quickly and decisively to whether men feel capable and successful, causing changes in mood, mental health and resilience. In *Part 8: How to Talk to Him*, we'll return to this knowledge and use it to great effect, introducing a simple strategy that makes it easy to have natural, supportive conversations with men in all kinds of situations.

There's another important side to this conversation. In workshops where we discuss testosterone and football results, people sometimes raise the issue of domestic abuse linked to football matches. You may have heard the terrifying news that research shows domestic abuse increases on days when the sports teams play — especially during football fixtures, and particularly when teams lose.

In 2021, the *Centre for Economic Performance (CEP)* in the UK published an analysis of data from Greater Manchester Police, covering nearly 800 local football game days. They found that although incidents of domestic abuse rose on match days, this rise was closely linked to alcohol consumption. Where the perpetrator had not been drinking, there was no increase in abuse over and above a non-game day. [92]

By analysing the time of the calls, CEP found that emergency calls slightly decreased when matches began but rose steadily afterwards, peaking around 10 hours after the game. In the words of Ria Ivandic, lecturer in political economy at the University of Oxford and a research economist at CEP:

"These results suggest that sporting events do not trigger domestic abuse by themselves, but rather through the excessive alcohol consumption that usually follows these events. Games scheduled at midday or afternoon enable perpetrators to start drinking early and continue throughout the day, leading to a peak in domestic abuse in the late evening by perpetrators who have been drinking. Delaying the start of the games until the evening and scheduling them on weekdays would help prevent a considerable amount of domestic abuse." [93]

While football, testosterone, and heightened emotion are often blamed, the evidence points more clearly to alcohol as the key driver. That's not to excuse abusive behaviour – nothing justifies it – but it's important we focus on the true risk factors if we want to prevent it.

Looking After Body & Mind: Strategies

Looking After Body & Mind is about male hormonal health. In this part of the book, we have explored how testosterone levels in men often reflect lifestyle factors. By dispelling the misconceptions surrounding health, we can support the men we care about to lead a testosterone-boosting lifestyle, greatly improving their physical, mental and metabolic health.

❏ Real food: reduce carbohydrates; increase natural fats

Modern dietary guidelines encourage men to base their meals on carbohydrates, choose low-fat options and avoid saturated fat.

There are many reasons I believe this kind of diet plays a central role in today's decline in testosterone in the men we care about: [94]

1. Reducing fat in a man's diet has been found to reduce his testosterone
2. In the long term, carbohydrate-based diets can contribute to insulin resistance which reduces testosterone production in men
3. In the short term, a large dose of sugar (specifically glucose) can significantly reduce testosterone in men for at least several hours
4. Since the introduction of the carbohydrate-based dietary guidelines, testosterone levels have sharply decreased
5. Ketogenic diets (low in carbohydrates, high in natural fat) quickly and consistently increase testosterone in men

The most powerful strategy for increasing testosterone quickly and naturally in men is to follow a low-carbohydrate diet that's based on real food (rather than ultra-processed food). Not only is this beneficial for testosterone levels, but it can lead to other big improvements to physical health, mental health, and energy levels.

I'm afraid the job of this section of the book isn't to give you a step-by-step meal plan for men, as what we eat should be personalised to each person's current health, goals, and level of activity. The aim here is to help you understand that many of the health issues men face today — including low testosterone — are linked to diet, and can often be improved with better food choices.

The *Public Health Collaboration (PHC)* is a UK registered charity dedicated to improving the health of the public and saving the NHS money at the same time. Founded by health and fitness experts and NHS doctors and whose practices have above average outcomes for their patients, the PHC's mission is:

"To empower, inspire and educate people that most chronic diseases can be prevented and reversed by maintaining good metabolic health through sustainable lifestyle changes." [95]

A big part of their approach is to coach their patients to eat fewer carbohydrates and processed food, and more "real" foods containing nutrients and natural fat. My Resources page links to their website where you will find:

- A simple guide to assess your metabolic health.
- Free, visual food charts ranking foods from:
    - "Low-Carbohydrate"
    - "Medium" and "High"
    - "Very High" and "Fake Food"
- Budgeting guidelines to ensure a healthy diet is accessible to all.

The PHC's visualisations make it easier for people to picture which foods will raise their blood sugar levels, and to make informed decisions around their diet. Nowhere in their leaflets does it suggest that a "Real Food" diet will increase testosterone in men, but by improving metabolic health, it will. After months of research and speaking to nutritionists familiar with low-carb diets, the diet that boosted my testosterone from 20.4 to 29.7 nmol/L was almost identical to the diet recommended by the PHC. It would have saved me a lot of time if I'd found them first!

The only significant difference between my diet and the PHC's "Real Food" diet was that I also avoided mint and liquorice and started adding natural ginger to my food, because I'd found several human and animal studies to suggest that this would increase my testosterone levels by reducing inflammation. [96] [97] [98] [99] [100]

If you have a medical condition, mental health condition, or take medication, it's very important you work with your doctor if you begin a low-carbohydrate diet or fasting. Improving your metabolic health with a low-carbohydrate diet can address the underlying causes of many health issues, which can quickly leave you over-medicated. The University of Manitoba and the *British Journal of General Practice* have published helpful guides you can share with your doctor, on how to safely reduce and discontinue your medications when you get into fat-burning mode (ketosis). Both are available on the resources page of my website - TheMensCoach.co.uk/resources under "Tools for Healthcare Practitioners".

While low-carbohydrate diets are quite simple for men, there are more considerations for women. The 2 books I recommend for women are *Fast Like a Girl* by Dr Mindy Pelz, and *Hungry Women* by Pauline Cox.

While diet seems to have the biggest impact on testosterone levels in men, there are other links in the chain that also need to be in place — and that's what the other strategies here are designed to address.

❑ Sleep: 7-8 hours per day

Sleep and testosterone seem to have a two-way relationship. Low testosterone in men has been linked to worse sleep quality, including more waking at night. But quality sleep may also play a key role in testosterone production. This means men can become stuck in a vicious cycle of poor sleep and low testosterone. In my work, I often find that men who say they struggle to sleep turn out to have low testosterone. [101]

There are several small experiments that have monitored testosterone levels in men during sleep. They found that testosterone levels in men rise with each hour of sleep, and decrease with each waking hour. By depriving men of sleep, the experiments caused testosterone levels to significantly reduce. [102] [103]

A 2018 study on lifestyle and testosterone levels in men suggests that each single missed hour of sleep is associated with a testosterone reduction roughly equivalent to 12 years of ageing! On their own, neither of these reductions would be disastrous, but it suggests that sleep plays a much larger role in testosterone levels than ageing. My own experience is when men focus more on getting 7–8 hours of sleep, it can have a very positive impact on testosterone levels. [104]

I once worked with a man who called me in a panic as he had received an extremely low testosterone test result. He had tested at 9 a.m., as his clinic recommended. But the clinic hadn't realised that he was an ambulance driver and would be returning from a busy night shift at 9 a.m.! After we spoke, he decided to focus on his sleep for a few days and then test again within 2 hours of waking. After prioritising good sleep for a few days, he had a much healthier testosterone level.

How much sleep we need is a hotly debated topic, but multiple studies have suggested that men who sleep 7–8 hours in every 24 seem to live the longest. I find they also have the healthiest testosterone levels. [105]

But poor sleep is a difficult cycle to break. Here are some techniques that have worked well for many of my clients who were previously struggling with sleep:

1. Have a set 'getting up' time, rather than a set bed time.
2. Exercise in the first few hours of waking, rather than before bed.
3. Write down and complete a goal every day, giving a sense of achievement.

❏ Exercise: 150 minutes / week

Not only is exercise important for testosterone production, it's essential for positive mental health. The NHS recommend that all adults should aim to: [106]

- do at least 150 minutes of moderate intensity activity a week or 75 minutes of vigorous intensity activity a week

- do strengthening activities that work all the major muscle groups on at least 2 days a week
- spread exercise evenly over 4 to 5 days a week, or every day
- reduce time spent sitting or lying down and break up long periods of not moving with some activity

In 2023, an analysis involving 128,119 people found that 150 minutes of exercise a week is significantly more effective than antidepressant medication or talking therapy when it comes to the treatment of depression, stress, and anxiety. This doesn't take away from the effectiveness of antidepressants or talking therapy, but I believe it does put it in perspective. [107]

This is important to know because if you know a man who goes to the doctor because he's feeling depressed, it's very possible that he will leave that appointment with a referral to therapy and a prescription for depressants (just like Brad did). But he might not know that the single most effective thing he can do is something that has no waiting list, no lead times, and no nasty side effects: to put on some comfortable shoes and be physically active for 20 minutes.

If you're wondering what counts as exercise, it's anything that *"will raise your heart rate, and make you breathe faster and feel warmer. One way to tell if you're working at a moderate intensity level is if you can still talk, but not sing."* Examples from the NHS include brisk walking, riding a bike, dancing, tennis, hiking, and pushing a lawn mower. [108]

The NHS suggests that *"Vigorous intensity activity makes you breathe hard and fast. If you're working at this level, you will not be able to say more than a few words without pausing for breath. In general, 75 minutes of vigorous intensity activity a week can give similar health benefits to 150 minutes of moderate intensity activity."* Examples include running, swimming, cycling quickly or up hills, skipping and sports like football.

Exercise at different times of the day also seems to have slightly different benefits. It's suggested that exercise in the first few hours after waking is best for concentration, calmness, and sleep; exercising later in the day (and after eating) is better for performance and reducing insulin resistance.

Exercising at any time of the day has a similar effect on weight loss. But the worst kind of exercise is no exercise at all! If in doubt, be physically active at whatever time of day you can fit it into your schedule. [109]

I find that men have a tendency to focus on weightlifting, but it's the intense workouts (like HIIT sessions) that increase testosterone the most, especially when the workout includes legs.

Be mindful, however. It's possible to overdo it. When I work with men who are doing intense exercise for several hours a day (perhaps training for a fitness challenge), they have low testosterone levels while they are training intensely. But once they have completed the challenge and re-introduce some rest days, testosterone usually bounces back, providing all the other lifestyle factors are in place.

❏ Vitamin D3: sunlight, supplements, natural fat

Vitamin D isn't just a vitamin, it's also used by your body as a hormone. The most helpful form is called vitamin D3. It supports strong bones, a healthy immune system, muscle strength, and brain health. [110]

There are several reasons to believe that D3 may also be important for testosterone production. A study of 54 men with low vitamin D found that taking a daily vitamin D supplement was associated with an increased level of testosterone. Those who were given a placebo did not have any increase. The study suggests that increasing vitamin D levels could increase testosterone levels in men with low vitamin D. [111]

Our ancestors probably didn't have to worry about vitamin D3 because of their lifestyle and the amount of time they spent outside. Your body is extremely efficient at making vitamin D3: you just need sunshine and cholesterol. You can also absorb vitamin D3 by eating fatty fish – rainbow trout, sockeye salmon, and sardines. But it should be wild fish, because farmed fish don't get the sunlight they need to make as much D3. [112][113]

Unfortunately, low-fat diets and indoor living means that many of us are now D3 deficient. And so many healthcare providers around the world suggest that most adults would benefit from D3 supplements.

What's more, because D3 is fat-soluble, your body can't absorb it unless you have enough fat with it. A study had participants take a high-dose vitamin D3 supplement with either a fat-rich meal or a high-carb, low-fat meal. Over the following two weeks, those who took the supplement with the fat-rich meal saw a 26% increase in D3 levels, while those who had the low-fat, high-carb meal actually had a 7% decrease in vitamin D. This shows that supplements alone may not be enough to compensate for diet. [114]

A ketogenic diet, which is naturally high in fat, seems to enhance this effect: in a study of 38 men, D3 levels increased by an average of 90% after 12 weeks. I don't know whether the participants were taking vitamin D supplements at the same time, but that's an impressive increase either way. [115]

❏ Reduce / stop drinking alcohol

Many people assume that alcohol and testosterone go hand in hand, but they don't get along at all. In an analysis of 2,296 men, each single alcoholic drink was associated with a testosterone reduction roughly equivalent to 6 years of ageing. [116]

Near the beginning of this book, I mentioned a study linking a testosterone level of 15.1 nmol/L and below with heart attacks in men aged 46 to 89. That same study of men aged found that **most (62%) heavy drinkers in the study had testosterone levels below 10.4 nmol/L**. [117]

Long term alcohol use seems to reduce testosterone in men. Men with testosterone are much more likely to be depressed. And what do depressed men often like to do? Often it's to drink alcohol - creating a vicious cycle. It's important we all know when to have some time without drinking alcohol.

In my coaching programme, I ask all participants to complete 21 days of sobriety, combined with daily goal-setting and 7 a.m. accountability calls. The benefits are twofold. First, time without alcohol naturally boosts testosterone, motivation, and decision-making (more on that in Part 5: Having Adventures). Second, because drinking is so socially ingrained — especially around holidays — abstaining for three weeks forces men to practice saying no, even when others encourage them to "*just have one.*" This strengthens determination, which ripples through all areas of life. This structured approach is called the Tough 21 Protocol and forms the foundation of my coaching method.

❏ Watch team wins

Many people are reluctant to give this a go because it seems too simple to be true. However, I have been told by many women that this strategy has transformed the atmosphere in their house on days where sports teams are playing.

If you have male sports fans at home, suggest that – if their team loses a meaningful match – they then watch an impressive past performance.

This beats the post-match blues for me and has worked very well for many men I have worked with. Some men already do this without realising – I'm regularly told during workshops that "our TV box is full of recordings of matches that his team has won!" So why not turn this into a structured strategy to improve the hormones, mood and (potentially) the mental health in the men we care about?

Ultimately, our aim is to help the men we care about prioritise the self-maintenance habits that make the biggest difference. I find that framing the conversation around testosterone engages men, motivates them to take action, and also gives them a tangible way to track their progress. And while nothing in this section is an alternative to professional help, professional support should not be seen as a replacement for Looking After Body & Mind.

ENDNOTES

1. R1555: The Public Health Collaboration (Accessed 2025). "How to Measure Metabolic Health." PHCUK.org.
2. R1546: L Araújo et al (2019). "Prevalence of Optimal Metabolic Health in American Adults: National Health and Nutrition Examination Survey 2009–2016." Metabolic Syndrome and Related Disorders.
3. R1563: C Murdoch (2024). "Insulin Resistance Health Check." HealthShelf.org.
4. R444: A Perheentupa et al. (2013). "A cohort effect on serum testosterone levels in Finnish men." European Journal of Endocrinology.
5. R442: A-M Andersson et al. (2007). "Secular decline in male testosterone and sex hormone binding globulin serum levels in Danish population surveys." The Journal of Clinical Endocrinology & Metabolism.
6. R1391: P Trimpou et al. (2012). "Secular trends in sex hormones and fractures in men and women." European Journal of Endocrinology.
7. R443: T G Travison et al. (2007). "A population-level decline in serum testosterone levels in American men." The Journal of Clinical Endocrinology & Metabolism.
8. R1481: K Kahl (2020). "Testosterone levels show steady decrease among young US men." Urology Times.
9. R531: T W Kelsey et al. (2014). "A validated age-related normative model for male total testosterone shows increasing variance but no decline after age 40 years." PLOS One.
10. R1020: R DeFronzo et al. (2009). "Skeletal muscle insulin resistance is the primary defect in type 2 diabetes." Diabetes Care.
11. R709: V Giner et al. (2001). "Increased insulin resistance in salt sensitive essential hypertension." Journal of Human Hypertension.
12. R710: M Suzuki et al. (2000). "Association of insulin resistance with salt sensitivity and nocturnal fall of blood pressure." Hypertension.
13. R1483: C Zhang et al. (2020). "Molecular mechanisms of hepatic insulin resistance in nonalcoholic fatty liver disease and potential treatment strategies." Pharmacological Research.
14. R1004: G Reaven (1991). "Insulin resistance and compensatory hyperinsulinemia: Role in hypertension, dyslipidemia, and coronary heart disease." American Heart Journal.
15. R769: J A Hamer et al. (2019). "Brain insulin resistance: A treatment target for cognitive impairment and anhedonia in depression." Experimental Neurology.
16. R1404: A Miola et al. (2023). "Insulin resistance in bipolar disorder: A systematic review of illness course and clinical correlates." Journal of Affective Disorders.
17. R1405: S Rege (2024). "Brain insulin resistance: Mechanisms, neuropsychiatric implications and therapeutic frontiers." Psych Scene Hub.
18. R1406: S Alves et al. (2025). "Insulin signaling disruption exacerbates memory impairment and seizure susceptibility in an epilepsy model with Alzheimer's disease-like pathology." Neurology and Preclinical Neurological Studies.
19. R1507: A Vikram et al. (2010). "Insulin-resistance and benign prostatic hyperplasia: the connection" European Journal of Pharmacology.

20 R1562: J Trussell et al (2007). "Erectile dysfunction: does insulin resistance play a part?." Fertility and Sterility.
21 R1094: L Ramírez-Martínez et al. (2024). "The potential for ketogenic diets to control glucotoxicity, hyperinsulinemia, and insulin resistance to improve fertility in women with polycystic ovary syndrome." Clinical and Experimental Obstetrics & Gynecology.
22 R1058: F Toledo et al. (2021). "Understanding the contribution of insulin resistance to the risk of pancreatic cancer." The American Journal of Gastroenterology.
23 R1103: A Mandel (2023). "Insulin resistance symptoms." News Medical.
24 There's a lot of research showing that conditions like depression, heart disease, type 2 diabetes, high blood pressure, schizophrenia, and even enlarged prostate are linked to a higher risk of suicide. If you'd like to read them, you will find numerous studies on PubMed or Google Scholar. Here, I'm just focusing on sharing sources for the link between insulin resistance and suicide.
25 R1098: H Koponen et al. (2015). "Association between suicidal behaviour and impaired glucose metabolism in depressive disorders." BMC Psychiatry.
26 R1081: Y Lee et al. (2018). "Association between insulin resistance and depression in the general Korean population: Cross sectional findings from the national health and nutrition examination survey." Korean Journal of Psychosomatic Medicine.
27 R1407: Y Choo et al. (2021). "Sociodemographic factors, health behaviors, and biological indicators associated with suicide mortality among young adults in South Korea: A nationwide cohort study among 15 million men and women." The Journal of Clinical Psychiatry.
28 R1408: J Chang et al. (2013). "Metabolic syndrome and the risk of suicide: A community-based integrated screening samples cohort study." Psychosomatic Medicine.
29 R1002: N Pitteloud et al. (2005). "Increasing insulin resistance is associated with a decrease in leydig cell testosterone secretion in men." The Journal of Clinical Endocrinology & Metabolism.
30 R507: K Ottarsdottir et al. (2018). "The association between serum testosterone and insulin resistance: a longitudinal study." Endocrine Connections.
31 R1484: P Rao et al. (2013). "Testosterone and insulin resistance in the metabolic syndrome and T2DM in men." Nature Reviews Endocrinology.
32 Low testosterone being brought on by insulin resistance is called "metabolic hypogonadism". I don't use this term very often, because almost no one has heard of it. But that's really what Looking After Body & Mind is trying to address.
33 R672: National Confidential Inquiry into Suicide and Safety in Mental Health (NCISH) (2021). "Suicide by middle-aged men." The University of Manchester.
34 R1290: S Kersten (2001). "Mechanisms of nutritional and hormonal regulation of lipogenesis." EMBO reports.
35 R1521: NHS (Accessed 2025). "The eatwell guide." nhs.uk.
36 R609: NHS Inform Scotland (2023). "Food labelling." nhsinform.scot.
37 R491: Public Health Collaboration (2023). "Dr David Unwin's sugar infographics." phcuk.org.

38 R1231: K Catalano et al. (2014). "Insulin resistance induced by hyperinsulinemia coincides with a persistent alteration at the insulin receptor tyrosine kinase domain." PLOS One.
39 R1232: H Cen et al. (2021). "Transcriptomic analysis of human and mouse muscle during hyperinsulinemia demonstrates insulin receptor downregulation as a mechanism for insulin resistance." bioRxiv.
40 R1539: L M Caronia et al (2012). 'Abrupt decrease in serum testosterone levels after an oral glucose load in men: implications for screening for hypogonadism.' Clinical Endocrinology.
41 Each medium (500ml) bottle of Lucozade Original contains 39.6 grams of glucose. R1545: Waitrose & Partners (Accessed 2025). "Lucozade Energy Drink Original (500ml)." Waitrose.com.
42 R1009: D Whitehill (2019). "Lifestyle based remission in type 2 diabetes: implications for clinical practice." University of Manitoba.
43 R1321: C Murdoch et al (2019). "Adapting diabetes medication for low carbohydrate management of type 2 diabetes: a practical guide." British Journal of General Practice.
44 R913: V Gershuni et al. (2018). "Nutritional ketosis for weight management and reversal of metabolic syndrome." Current Nutrition Reports.
45 R1490: I Meira et al. (2019). "Ketogenic diet and epilepsy: What we know so far." Frontiers in Neuroscience.
46 R1009: D Whitehill (2019). "Lifestyle based remission in type 2 diabetes: implications for clinical practice." University of Manitoba.
47 R1486: Public Health Collaboration (Accessed 2025). "Randomised controlled trials (RCTs): Comparing low-carb diets of less than 130g carbohydrate per day to low-fat diets of less than 35% fat of total calories." https://phcuk.org/evidence/rcts/.
48 R1147: A Danan et al. (2022). "The ketogenic diet for refractory mental illness: A retrospective analysis of 31 inpatients." Frontiers in Psychiatry.
49 R1094: L Ramírez-Martínez et al. (2024). "The potential for ketogenic diets to control glucotoxicity, hyperinsulinemia, and insulin resistance to improve fertility in women with polycystic ovary syndrome." Clinical and Experimental Obstetrics & Gynecology.
50 R1487: A Kiryttopoulos et al. (2025). "Successful application of dietary ketogenic metabolic therapy in patients with glioblastoma: a clinical study." Frontiers Nutrition.
51 R1488: M Phillips et al. (2020). "Managing metastatic thymoma with metabolic and medical therapy: A case report." Frontiers in Oncology.
52 R656: S L Vignera et al. (2020). "The ketogenic diet corrects metabolic hypogonadism and preserves pancreatic ß-cell function in overweight/obese men: a single-arm uncontrolled study." Endocrine.
53 R900: L Mongioi et al. (2020). "Effectiveness of a very low calorie ketogenic diet on testicular function in overweight/obese men." Nutrients.
54 R899: J Wilson et al. (2020). "Effects of ketogenic dieting on body composition, strength, power, and hormonal profiles in resistance training men." Journal of Strength and Conditioning Research.

55 R1496: C Furini et al. (2023). "Ketogenic state improves testosterone serum levels- results from a systematic review and meta-analysis." Endocrine.
56 To assess my heart health I monitored my triglyceride to HDL cholesterol ratio (often written as "TG:HDL ratio").
57 R1492: J Volek et al. (2021). "Alternative dietary patterns for Americans: Low-carbohydrate diets." Nutrients.
58 R1476: I Cooper et al. (2024). "Ketosis suppression and ageing (ketosage) part 2: The effect of suppressing ketosis on biomarkers associated with ageing, homa-ir, leptin, osteocalcin, and GLP-1, in healthy females." Biomedicines.
59 R1221: M Dehghan et al. (2017). "Associations of fats and carbohydrate intake with cardiovascular disease and mortality in 18 countries from five continents (PURE): a prospective cohort study." The Lancet.
60 R1410: S-T P W et al. (2010). "Meta-analysis of prospective cohort studies evaluating the association of saturated fat with cardiovascular disease." The American Journal of Clinical Nutrition.
61 R1411: M Jakobsen et al. (2010). "Intake of carbohydrates compared with intake of saturated fatty acids and risk of myocardial infarction: importance of the glycemic index." The American Journal of Clinical Nutrition.
62 R1297: A C Wood et al. (2011). "Dietary carbohydrate modifies the inverse association between saturated fat intake and cholesterol on very low-density lipoproteins." Lipid Insights.
63 R1382: A Astrup et al. (2020). "Saturated fats and health: A reassessment and proposal for food-based recommendations: JACC state-of-the-art review." Journal of the American College of Cardiology.
64 R824: J Whittaker et al. (2021). "Low-fat diets and testosterone in men: Systematic review and meta-analysis of intervention studies." The Journal of Steroid Biochemistry and Molecular Biology.
65 R825: C Wang et al. (2005). "Low-fat high-fiber diet decreased serum and urine androgens in men." The Journal of Clinical Endocrinology & Metabolism.
66 R826: E K Hämäläinen et a (1983). "Decrease of serum total and free testosterone during a low-fat high-fibre diet." Journal of Steroid Biochemistry.
67 R961: M Katan (1998). "Effect of low-fat diets on plasma high-density lipoprotein concentrations." The American Journal of Clinical Nutrition.
68 R1282: E Hämäläinen et al. (1983). "Decrease of serum total and free testosterone during a low-fat high-fibre diet." Journal of Steroid Biochemistry.
69 R1305: Public Health Collaboration (Accessed 2025). "RCTs Comparing Low-Carb Diets Of Less Than 130g Carbohydrate Per Day To Low-Fat Diets Of Less Than 35% Fat Of Total Calories." phcuk.org. This is not an article from a scientific journal but a meta-analysis of RCTs hosted on a website.
70 R1497: A Ferrari et al. (2025). "Nonvesicular cholesterol transport in physiology." The Journal of Clinical Investigation.
71 R1547: Biology Insights (2025). "Cholesterol Biosynthesis: How Your Body Produces Cholesterol." biologyinsights.com.

72 R1548: B Griffin et al (1994). "Role of plasma triglyceride in the regulation of plasma low density lipoprotein (LDL) subfractions: relative contribution of small, dense LDL to coronary heart disease risk." Atherosclerosis.
73 No single source can fully back up this statement, but studies comparing different lipid ratios suggest that TG:HDL and TC:HDL are good indicators of insulin sensitivity, heart health, and hormonal balance. ApoB:ApoA1 is also a useful ratio, but TG:HDL is (I think) the most useful because it is based on figures that are taken during a normal cholesterol test and also appears to be a proxy for LDL particle size, which can help us to understand whether LDL cholesterol is a problem or not.
74 R1198: NHS Inform (accessed 2024). "High cholesterol." NHSinform.scot.
75 R652: S-W Yi (2019). "Total cholesterol and all-cause mortality by sex and age: a prospective cohort study among 12.8 million adults." Scientific Reports.
76 By "3.5× more likely to die in the following 10 years" I am referring to the findings that men aged 45-54 with total cholesterol below 3.1 mmol/L had a hazard ratio (HR) of 3.39 vs 5.8 mmol/L - or 3.49 vs 6.9 mmol/L.
77 R1293: G He et al. (2021). "A nonlinear association of total cholesterol with all-cause and cause-specific mortality." Nutrition & Metabolism.
78 For example, in 2015 ischaemic heart disease accounted for 14.2% of deaths in UK men. R165: GOV.UK (2017). "Chapter 2: major causes of death and how they have changed." GOV.UK
79 R1412: J Neaton et al. (1992). "Serum cholesterol level and mortality findings for men screened in the multiple risk factor intervention trial." Archives of Internal Medicine.
80 R1413: G Lindberg et al. (1992). "Low serum cholesterol concentration and short term (sic.) mortality from injuries in men and women." The British Medical Journal.
81 R1402: L Ellison et al. (2001). "Low serum cholesterol concentration and risk of suicide." Epidemiology.
82 R251: D Blum (1997). "Sex on the Brain: The Biological Differences Between Men and Women." Penguin Books.
83 R138: A Booth et al. (1989). "Testosterone, and winning and losing in human competition." Hormones and Behavior.
84 R252: A Mazur, A Booth (1992). "Testosterone and Chess Competition." Social Psychology Quarterly.
85 R1560: D Longman et al (2018). "Tandem Androgenic and Psychological Shifts in Male Reproductive Effort Following a Manipulated "Win" or "Loss" in a Sporting Competition." Human Nature.
86 R253: C Suplee (1995). "Score one for the hormone team." Washington Post.
87 R946: P C Bernhardt et al. (1998). "Testosterone changes during vicarious experiences of winning and losing among fans at sporting events." Physiology & Behavior.
88 R705: D Carroll et al. (2002). "Admissions for myocardial infarction and World Cup football: database survey." The British Medical Journal.
89 R706: W Kirkup et al. (2003). "A matter of life and death: population mortality and football results." Journal of Epidemiology & Community Health.

90 R745: L Toubiana et al. (2001). "French cardiovascular mortality did not increase during 1996 European football championship." The British Medical Journal.
91 R706: W Kirkup et al. (2003).
92 R136: R Ivandic et al. (2021). "Football, alcohol and domestic abuse." Centre for Economic Performance.
93 R1558: Centre for Economic Performance (2021). "Alcohol, not emotions, responsible for domestic abuse rise after football matches: Domestic abuse risk could be reduced by later kick-offs and weekday matches." cep.lse.ac.uk.
94 For sources to support these statements, see Looking After Body & Mind: The Science.
95 R1494: Public Health Collaboration (Accessed 2025). "About." PHCUK.org.
96 R749: V Kumar (2008). "Spearmint induced hypothalamic oxidative stress and testicular anti-androgenicity in male rats – altered levels of gene expression, enzymes and hormones." Food and Chemical Toxicology.
97 R914: M Akdogan et al. (2004). "Effects of peppermint teas on plasma testosterone, follicle-stimulating hormone, and luteinizing hormone levels and testicular tissue in rats." Urology.
98 R750: D Aramani et al. (1999). "Reduction of serum testosterone in men by licorice." The New England Journal of Medicine.
99 R751: D Aramani et al. (2003). "Licorice consumption and serum testosterone in healthy man (sic)." Experimental and Clinical Endocrinology & Diabetes.
100 R570: S A Banihani (2018). "Ginger and testosterone." Biomolecules.
101 R241: E Barrett-Connor (2008). "The association of testosterone levels with overall sleep quality, sleep architecture, and sleep-disordered breathing." The Journal of Clinical Endocrinology and Metabolism.
102 R624: J Axelsson et al. (2005). "Effects of acutely displaced sleep on testosterone." The Journal of Clinical Endocrinology and Metabolism .
103 R604: R Leproult et al. (2011). "Effect of 1 week of sleep restriction on testosterone levels in young healthy men." JAMA.
104 R128: P Patel et al. (2018). "Impaired sleep is associated with low testosterone in us adult males: results from the national health and nutrition survey." Fertility and Sterility. - "On multivariate linear regression, we found serum testosterone decreased by 0.49 ng/dL per year of age (p = 0.04), 5.85 ng/dL per hour loss of sleep (p = < 0.01), 6.18 ng/dL per unit of body mass index (BMI) increase (p = < 0.01) and 2.99 ng/dL per each increase in alcoholic beverage (p = < 0.01)"
105 R342: K Jung et al. (2013). "Gender differences in nighttime sleep and daytime napping as predictors of mortality in older adults: The Rancho Bernardo Study." Sleep Medicine.
106 R249: NHS (2023). "Physical activity guidelines for adults aged 19 to 64." NHS.uk.
107 R258: B Singh et al. (2023). "Effectiveness of physical activity interventions for improving depression, anxiety and distress: an overview of systematic reviews." British Journal of Sports Medicine.
108 R249: NHS (2023). "Physical activity guidelines for adults aged 19 to 64." NHS.uk.
109 R1114: R Parke (2024). "What's the best time of day to work out – before or after work?" Newhorizoncrossfit.co.uk

110 The term 'vitamin D' actually refers to several related compounds. When UVB light from sunlight hits your skin, it turns cholesterol into cholecalciferol (vitamin D_3). Wild fatty fish also contain vitamin D_3, which is why cholecalciferol is classed as a vitamin. Your liver turns this into calcidiol, a pre-hormone that circulates in your blood, and your kidneys turn that into calcitriol, the active hormone. I also find the names confusing.

111 R134: S Pilz, S Frisch, H Koertke et al. (2011). "Effect of vitamin D supplementation on testosterone levels in men." Hormone and Metabolic Research.

112 R1227: J MacDonald (2019). "How does the body make vitamin D from sunlight?" JSTOR Daily.

113 R600: WebMD (Accessed 2025). "Foods high in vitamin D3." webmd.com.

114 R1228: F Raimundo et al. (2011). "Effect of high- versus low-fat meal on serum 25-hydroxyvitamin D Levels after a single oral dose of vitamin D: A single-blind, parallel, randomized trial." International Journal of Endocrinology.

115 R900: L Mongioi et al. (2020). "Effectiveness of a very low calorie ketogenic diet on testicular function in overweight/obese men." Nutrients.

116 R128: P Patel et al (2018). "Impaired sleep is associated with low testosterone in us adult males: results from the national health and nutrition survey." Fertility and Sterility.

117 R561: C Swartz et al (1987). "Low Serum Testosterone and Myocardial Infarction in Geriatric Male Inpatients." Journal of the American Geriatrics Society.

PART 4

PROTECTING THE CAVE

*"Security is not having things,
it's handling things"*

— Susan Jeffers

Protecting the Cave	
Signs of stress	• Feeling *overwhelmed* • Feeling *hopeless* or *ashamed* • Financial uncertainty • Relationship insecurity • Feeling *like a burden*

Gary's story

The rain beat down loudly on the wooden roof of Gary's office, generating a loud humming noise that lasted for our entire 2-hour coaching call. Built in the garden of his family home, Gary described his office as *"just a big shed, really."* But I could clearly see the care and skill that had gone into it, just from it being the backdrop to our Zoom call.

"That's the one thing about me, mate," Gary said. *"I'm good with my hands. I can build things like this."* I assured him that I was confident he had many more skills too.

While we talked through The ALPHA Framework together, Gary was generally talkative and light-hearted. He was fascinated by the link between testosterone and mental health, and shared how he had always found sleep and exercise to be key to his wellbeing. The exception was when we talked through Protecting the Cave. Throughout this section, he was quiet and thoughtful. He stopped asking questions and began staring out of the window into his rainy garden.

I wondered whether Protecting the Cave would come up during our Future Call exercise. It did.

Gary's Future Call

Ryan: Ring-ring! Ring-ring! Ah, Gary. I wasn't expecting your call – how are you doing?

Gary: Yes, mate, good thanks. Actually, things are different now. They're actually better than they have been in years. The family is good. The business is profitable again. And that's just really taken the pressure off the situation. It's so different from what it was when we first met one year ago today...

[Gary continued sharing with me how he had built up his construction business. We talked around the other Dimensions of The ALPHA Framework until I was happy he was in a problem-solving mode, then I asked him the important questions at the end of the exercise:]

Ryan: Cast your mind back to when we had that very first Zoom call together one year ago... At the time, what was the main thing that was holding you back?

Gary: It was money, mate. Essentially, when we met online last year, I had just lost a big contract that my business relied on. Without that contract, the business lost most of the income, but we still had the same salaries and overheads to cover. I didn't want to lay anyone off, so, to save the company, I stopped taking any salary or any dividends out. I didn't want it to fold. I inherited the company from my dad, and it would kill him to see it fail. So my family had no money coming in, but still we kept spending like it was the good old days. I can't tell you how stressful it was; I felt like I had put my own family in a sinking boat. Then I started having these thoughts, mate. I started to realise that… All the debts were in my name, so they would die with me. Plus my life insurance would kick in, taking care of Emily and the kids. As soon as I realised that… Mate, I couldn't stop thinking about it. About ending it all… Each time I was on site working, it was a thought in the back of my mind. It just seemed like the solution to everything, mate…

Ryan: What did you do to overcome those thoughts about killing yourself?

Gary: You said it in one sentence, mate: "*Protecting the Cave.*" That's what I wasn't doing. I was doing the talking groups that Emily wanted me to go to, but we were just talking round and round in circles. I'm sure it works for others, but it didn't work for me. It actually made it worse, because the guys there used to comment on how nice my house was, or how nice Emily's car was. All I could see was the financial pressure building behind the scenes. But during our call last year, I realised that I wasn't actually addressing the underlying problem: we were spending the same as we were when I had an income. I had to fix it. I had to Protect the Cave, mate, for the sake of my family.

Ryan: Well done, Gary. You've had an amazing year, but I want to know: what has been the single best thing you've done all year?

Gary: … I set aside one day every week to work on replacing the lost contract. Yes, that's what I did. And it was great because when we did replace the lost contract, I still kept that day aside for networking and business development. It made the business better because we always had a pipeline of new opportunities. Just setting that time aside to tackle the problem was so important to me. It gave me hope that the situation could be addressed. I needed to feel that, mate. I needed to feel that there was something practical I could do. And that I didn't need to… do anything drastic…

Ryan: If I had a time machine, and you could send a message back in time to be delivered to Gary at the end of his first coaching session one year ago, what would you say to him? What did he need to hear at the time?

Gary: Oh, that's a great question. I would say to him... *"Hang in there. Remind yourself who you are, and what you are capable of. Reflect on what you've overcome in the past. These current challenges are all surmountable: identify the problems and fix them."*

[At this point, Gary tilted his head back, to stop tears from running down his face. He breathed two big sighs of relief.]

Gary: I'm sorry, mate. Can I add one more thing to the message? There's something else he... I... needed to know one year ago... *"You are actually an asset... To your team... To your business... To your family. So you just hang in there and keep chipping away at the money situation. You need to protect that cave. And to do that, your family need you to be here."*

Ryan: It's been an absolute honour seeing what you've achieved over the past year, Gary, but I want to know... Cast your mind back to that first coaching session we had a year ago. When you left the coaching call, what was the very first thing you did that got this amazing year off to a great start?

Gary: Hmm. Another good question... I went and sat down with Emily. And I told her where we were at. I told her about the finances, and my plan to fix them. And I told her about my thoughts, and my plan to fix them too. Then we made a list of all the ways I contribute to the family, and to the kids, and we put a value next to them all. And when that value exceeded the amount of money my family would get if I died, I started to see myself as an asset again. I kept that list in my pocket all year. At first, I would pull it out and read it when I was having the thoughts. But by the end of the year, it was enough just to have the letter in my van.

Ryan: Well done, mate. You've had an amazing year and it's been my honour to watch you achieve so much. I know there were times where you made use of the expertise of others – friends, family, charities and experts that helped with financial planning – but ultimately *YOU*

> made this happen. You realised what needed to be addressed, and you then went and addressed it. And I want you to know that your family are proud of you, your team are proud of you, I'm proud of you, and you should be proud of yourself.
>
> Gary: You don't know how much that means, mate.
>
> Ryan: Look, I have to go now, but it was great catching up.
>
> Gary: Thank you, mate.
>
> Ryan: Bye, Gary.
> *BEEP*

After the Future Call, Gary and I created a plan to keep himself safe, and he promised to speak to a charity that specialises in debt if the thoughts returned. But he didn't need to. When he shared his experiences with his partner, Emily, she asked him what he needed. They committed to a monthly "finances date" – a whole evening dedicated to reviewing what they spent last month and adjusting their plan moving forwards.

Three months after our first coaching session, Gary called me to tell me that he had replaced the lost contract, but that he was keeping his Tuesdays reserved solely for networking and business development. When I asked him for his main insight from the whole experience, he said it was that he needed to stay open and honest with his partner Emily. Their "finance dates" had become the foundation of their new relationship with money, and with eachother. Tackling the challenges head on on had been the most powerful tool in overcoming his thoughts about suicide.

Protecting the Cave is about the things men can do for their sense of security.

Protecting the Cave: The science

Financial security and male mental health

There are 2 main sources of security that seem to matter the most to men: the first is *financial security*.

I started to take an interest in financial security and male mental health in 2020, when I was reading a study that had just been published in *Annals of General Psychiatry*. It was a study of 5,514 people over the age of 60, living in rural China. I know that's strangely specific, but what interested me about this study was that it compared gender differences around suicide.[1]

The people who took part in the study answered questions relating to their marital status, education level, health, debt, stress of daily lives, family relationships, and negative life events. These factors were then compared with whether or not people were having thoughts about suicide. In men in the study, debt was the strongest factor found to be associated with suicide. In fact, men with debt had **6.5× higher odds** of having thoughts about suicide, versus those without debt. (To put that into perspective, having *chronic health issues* like cancer or high blood pressure had 2.5× increased odds.)

Even after taking compounding factors into consideration, debt remained the strongest factor associated with thoughts about suicide in men, alongside being illiterate.

In women, the biggest factors were different: stressful daily life, being illiterate, and negative life events. Having debt didn't make the top 3. The study concluded that:

"There was a significant gender difference towards suicidal ideation among rural elderly in Shandong, China."

Of course, this study only included elderly people in China, so it's not necessarily representative of people elsewhere. But it made me wonder whether there was more evidence of a connection between financial security and suicide in men, or whether this was an exception.

It turns out, this link doesn't only apply to men in rural China.

Analysis by the UK's National Confidential Inquiry into Suicide and Safety in Mental Health (a report I reference multiple times in this book) suggests that as many as 57% of middle-aged UK men who die from suicide are experiencing economic challenges at the time of their death. That's the majority. Nearly 1 in 3 (30%) of middle-aged men who died from suicide were unemployed at the time of their death. And research by Samaritans has suggested that unemployment plays a key role in driving suicide in middle-aged men. [2] [3]

Staying with the UK for just a moment longer, data from the Office for National Statistics shows that the most likely socioeconomic group to die from suicide are men who are long-term unemployed or have never worked. Men in this group are 2.3× more likely to die from suicide than the average UK man, and 6.7× more likely than the average UK woman. [4]

In 2025, non-profit organisation Equimundo published their *State of American Men 2025* report. This was a survey of 2,454 people – 75% of which were men. Among other things, they found: [5]

- Economic anxiety is at the forefront of American men's minds.
- Men who face financial insecurity are 16.3× more likely to have had thought about suicide in the past 2 weeks (compared to 7.3× in women).
- 86% of men agreed with the statement "*In my opinion being a man is: providing for my family.*" (This was the most common answer, followed by "being a friend" and "being strong" – both 82%).
- 77% of women list "provider" as their top trait a man should have.

But what if the trend goes even further than the UK and the US?

In 2021, a team from the University of Padova in Italy compared 26 years of economic data and suicide statistics from 175 countries (that's about 90% of all the world's countries). They analysed high, low, and middle-income countries, from Afghanistan, Albania, and Algeria to Zambia and Zimbabwe. [6]

This unprecedented amount of economic and suicide data showed that as economies grow, suicide rates reduce. As economies shrink, suicide rates increase. And when unemployment rises, the gap between male and female suicide rates gets wider, with males being worse affected. This aligns with the findings of the other studies I mentioned: men appear to be much more vulnerable to financial insecurity – especially debt and unemployment – than women are.

This enormous study of worldwide data concluded with the words: *"Males who have lost their jobs in adulthood are those at higher risk of suicide and to whom financial support measures should be delivered in a timely manner."*

The article also contained an interesting suggestion, aimed at saving lives by giving financial support to those who have just lost their job:

"[...] Delivering 1000 US dollars to 500 people at high risk of suicide, with the prediction of saving at least 1 life, would economically cost less than 1 death by suicide (which is estimated to cost, directly and indirectly, at least 500,000 US dollars); in addition to the incommensurable human cost of losing a life to suicide."

But would it actually work that way? It seems very clear that financial security is important to male mental health. But does increasing financial security *improve* male mental health?

That's what we're going to look at next.

How improving financial security impacts male mental health

In 2016, Bristol was 1 of 8 UK regions with high rates of suicide awarded funding to address it. Charity Second Step knew that around 3 in 4 deaths from suicide are men. They had also identified that the rate of male suicide was falling, until the 2008 financial crisis and the following recession – highlighting that men are particularly vulnerable to economic pressures. Second Step created a service for men that would help them to address their thoughts about suicide and their debt, financial, housing, or employment issues. They called it the Hope project. [7]

Hope's team was a combination of:

- Project Workers – trained to provide a non-judgemental, solution-focussed form of therapy.
- Advice Workers – those with specific qualifications and experience to offer the men advice to address their financial issues.

A highly practical form of support, but was it effective?

A study was carried out to measure the impact of this support. During the study period, 413 men used the Hope project, with 80 completing the before and after questionnaires needed for the study. The results showed that:

After attending the Hope project, the number of men who were still having thoughts about suicide had reduced by 55%. And the severity of their depression (measured by a PHQ-9 questionnaire) was down by 49%. [8]

What an amazing improvement. To put it in perspective, this is the kind of improvement that majority-female groups typically show from CBT talking therapy, suggesting that tackling financial issues may be just as effective for depressed men as talking therapy is for depressed women. [9]

The experiences of men who used the Hope Project bring these results to life. Here are three quotes from Jackson et al.'s 2022 study published in *BMC Psychiatry*:

"When I first met up with (Hope Project worker) I was determined that life was at the end and I was fed-up and she turned it around. Like I couldn't get a bank account and she got me a bank account, came into the bank and helped me out, and if she weren't there I wouldn't have got it because I didn't have the relevant ID. I blow everything up into a really big problem and she cut it down into digestible chunks, if you like to call it that, and helped me through all of it. It's been great."

"To cut a long story short if it weren't for The Hope Project and (name) I would not have made it back out through the rabbit hole, I was done. And I can't thank the organisation enough because at the end of the day I've had several friends who've

committed suicide which is a terrible thing but what I know for one thing is sure if they were being given the same amount of help which I was given I'm sure that some of them would still be alive today that's how important The Hope Project is. I mean to cut a long story short, The Hope Project saves lives (original emphasis) that's a fact"

"They sorted my life out, I don't know what else I could say, my life at the time, I had my money slashed to bits which I don't know how I survived plus I felt myself sinking into depression. Between them, in completely different ways, (Project worker) and (Advice worker) have put me back on track. I don't know where I was going, I really don't, I wasn't sleeping, I wasn't eating, I was a bit of a mess. They certainly helped me."

This is support focused not just on **talking about problems**, but on actively **solving them**. The words of the men share how much these practical steps improved their mental health and often kept them alive, by helping them with the financial, housing, and employment challenges they were facing. I believe we can all learn a great deal from the Hope project.

Elsewhere in the world, a 13-year Australian study found that unemployment and underemployment (having a job, but not enough hours, pay, or use of their skills) were major contributors to suicide deaths during that period. Of the roughly 32,000 suicides recorded, about 1 in 5 were linked to people not having enough work — with over 3,000 deaths tied to unemployment and another 3,000 to underemployment. The researchers concluded that policies aiming for full employment should be considered an essential part of any national suicide prevention strategy. [10]

In my experience, when men start to see themselves as a financial burden, they can believe that the best way to tackle the issue is to get rid of the burden, i.e. themselves. Rather than spending time debating whether this is from societal pressures or a biological predisposition, I think it would be better for everyone if we simply equipped men with the support and problem-solving skills they need for their financial security. This would have many benefits, one of which is fewer male suicides.

To summarise what we've explored so far:

- Financial security is strongly associated with male mental health.
- Lack of financial security is a key driver of suicide in men, especially unemployment, debt, and homelessness.
- Tackling these financial issues has been found to improve male mental health and can address the underlying cause of thoughts of suicide in some men.

Alongside financial security, there is another form of security that's particularly important to male mental health.

Relationship security.

Relationship security and male mental health

Relationship breakdown seems to impact men and women in different ways. Several studies have found that relationship breakdown greatly increases the risk of suicide in men, more so than women.

In 2000, a large US study investigated how marital status, gender, and suicide might be related. The study found that divorced people have higher rates of suicide than married people. But when they split the data by gender, they found that increased rate of suicide was driven by men; in women, divorce was not associated with significantly higher suicide rates. [11]

The article, published in *Journal of Epidemiology & Community Health* suggested that *"combining men and women in the same models could produce misleading results."*

A slightly older study looked at deaths from suicide in Queensland Australia, and found that:

- Men who were recently separated (but not yet divorced) were **6× more likely to die from suicide** than married men. This was higher amongst younger men.
- Divorce also increased suicide risk in men, but not as much as the early separation.

- **Being married was a protective factor for men**, especially those aged 30–54.
- Men may be particularly vulnerable to the emotional impact of separation, especially when it involves interpersonal conflict.

In women, the findings were different. In women:

- Separation **did not** significantly increase risk of suicide.
- Divorce coming through increased suicide rates in women.
- Having children was a protective factor for women, but this faded as the children grew. [12]

One in-depth study of 100 cases of suicide in UK men classified the possible triggers of suicide and found that relationship breakdown appears to be the principal trigger of suicide in some men. [13]

So relationship breakdown seems to be a big issue, especially for men. But many studies and awareness campaigns focus on comparisons between married and separated men: what about men who have never married? I wanted to understand suicide rates in single men, because this could help clarify whether the increased rates in separated men are due to the separation itself or the broader loss of a relationship.

This data from the UK's Office for National Statistics shows the rates of male suicide based on relationship status from between 2011 and 2021: [14]

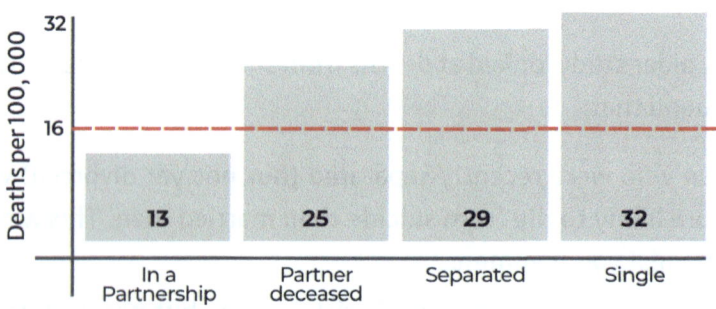

Adapted from R894: Office for National Statistics (2023). 'Sociodemographic inequalities in suicides in England and Wales: 2011 to 2021'. ons.gov.uk. Grouping based on ONS classifications: 'In a Partnership' (Married or in a registered same-sex partnership); 'Separated' (Either divorced or separated but still legally married or in a same-sex partnership); 'Single' (Never been married or in a same-sex civil partnership). Based on men aged 45. Dotted line represents average rate of male suicide for the period.

I picked men aged 45 for the table because they are the age group of men with the highest rate of suicide in the UK. But the data tells the same story for UK men in every age group.

At every age, UK men who are single have higher rates of suicide than separated men, higher even than men whose partner has died. To me, this suggests that the absence of a life partner — not just the event of separation — poses a great risk to men.

And so, being able to start and maintain a healthy life partnership is an important protective factor for male mental health. Of course, I am not suggesting that men *should* have a life partner — that's a choice for each individual. But for those who *want* a life partner, it's important to be able to overcome the obstacles preventing that from happening.

In coaching conversations, finding a partner is something that comes up a lot when I work with single men. There are various obstacles that prevent men from finding a partner. Some men often find themselves in the 'friend-zone'; others find themselves in a string of casual relationships but lose interest before something deeper develops. Overcoming such barriers is not something we are going to explore in this book, because this is not a book on dating and relationship strategies for men. What we will explore in this book, however, is what causes relationships to break down. And according to multiple sources, the main cause of relationship breakdown is communication breakdown.

In a heterosexual relationship, I believe that communication breakdown is made more likely by the hormone that is thought to connect us. Specifically, the ways it affects males and females in a totally different way.

Oxytocin: The hormone that bonds us

Oxytocin is a hormone that is essential for processes like breastfeeding and childbirth (where it brings on the contractions that make birth happen).

Outside of these vital obstetric functions, oxytocin also plays a massive role in everyday life. In female mammals, oxytocin protects against stress and also makes female mammals bond with their partner – and with other females, which is why it is often referred to as the "love" or "bonding" hormone. [15][16]

Oxytocin is released by intimacy: stroking, cuddling, hugging, kissing, crying or having sex. In other primates, it is released when they spend time grooming those closest to them. In humans, gossiping is also thought to release oxytocin, and sharing how you feel is thought to trigger oxytocin release, by strengthening social bonds. [17][18][19][20]

When it comes to oxytocin, the way we communicate and comfort one another matters. In 2012, a study published in *Evolution and Human Behavior* measured oxytocin and stress levels in 68 girls (average age of 10) who were given different forms of support after a stressful experience (the Trier Social Stress Test for Children or "TSST-C").[21] I have summarised this study as succinctly as I can, but the details in the original article are well worth reading.

After the stress test, the girls were divided into 4 groups:

- Group 1 were brought to their mothers, who could congratulate and comfort them in person for 15 minutes.
- Group 2 were given 15 minutes to rest alone, with no social interaction or support.
- Group 3 didn't meet their mothers, but had a 15-minute phone call with them.
- Group 4 also didn't meet their mothers, but had a 15-minute instant message conversation with them.

After receiving the various forms of support, the girls watched a video until their stress levels returned to normal. There were lots of processes in place to ensure the safety of the girls through the experiment, despite the stress.

Oxytocin and cortisol (a marker for stress) were measured before and multiple times after the TSST-C, allowing the researchers to track which forms of support were most effective. Thirty minutes after the stressful experience, here's how the hormones differed between the different groups:

- In group 1 (in-person support from mum), the girls had high levels of oxytocin and low levels of cortisol. They were feeling connected and not stressed.
- In group 2 (no social support) the girls had low levels of oxytocin and high levels of cortisol. They were feeling disconnected and stressed.

Probably neither of those results are a surprise to you. But here's where it gets interesting:

- In group 3 (phone call with mum), oxytocin was as high and cortisol was as low as the in-person support. Connected and not stressed.
- In group 4 (instant messaging with mum), oxytocin was low and cortisol was higher than any other group. Disconnected and stressed.

This suggests that it's the comforting sound of a loved one's voice – not their words – that triggers the release of oxytocin. If you've ever felt calmer just by hearing someone's voice, this could be why. The study concluded:

"Due to the prevalence of this [instant messaging] in society, it is worth noting that it does not appear to fulfil all of the same biological functions as other types of social exchange, such as vocal communication and in-person interactions. In terms of stress mediation and oxytocin release, instant messaging is no substitute for spoken language or direct, interpersonal interaction between mothers and daughters in middle childhood."

So, in women, oxytocin is this incredible hormone that enables birth, breastfeeding, and falling in love – all while protecting you from stress. All you need to do to release oxytocin is to be close to those you care about: touch, hug, cry, or talk about how you feel. Amazing!

Oxytocin is so central to female mental health that it can be logical to assume that if men were to do the same thing, it would have the same effect. After all, men have higher rates of suicide and men are less likely to talk about how they feel, therefore men must have higher rates of suicide **because** they don't talk about how they feel and get that lovely boost of oxytocin. On the surface it seems logical. But this is based on the assumption that oxytocin affects men in the same way as women.

Let's look next at whether it does.

Oxytocin: The hormone that divides us

I regularly hear people say that men talk less about how they feel because of how they were raised. But I think it's possible that biology plays a larger role in this than many people realise.

For decades, scientific research has hinted that the hormones in our blood may impact the way our brain is organised - particularly the parts of our brain that are associated with word choice and emotions. [22] [23]

Around adolescence – the same age boys are said to start closing up – oxytocin levels seem to start to decline in boys. One study of 90 people suggests that, by adulthood, men's oxytocin levels may be around one third the average level found in women. [24] [25]

Does that reduction in oxytocin make men less inclined to talk about emotions? Well, one experiment tested exactly that. 60 healthy men were invited to discuss a painful memory. But first, half were given a dose of oxytocin (by a nasal spray), and the other half were given a placebo. The researchers then evaluated the way that the men described their painful experiences. While the amount of factual information shared was similar in both groups, oxytocin was found to make men more willing to share their emotions. [26]

To me, this suggests that the lower levels of oxytocin in men might explain why men are less likely to talk about how they feel - at least in part. So does this mean that men need oxytocin even more than women? After all, they seem to have less of it.

Well, that depends on the answer to our next question: *Does oxytocin actually reduce stress in men?*

This might seem like an odd question to ask, but this question first popped into my head when I realised that the vast majority of the studies I had read about the amazing stress-reducing qualities of oxytocin were based on women and girls. My hunch turned out to be right: there are both human and animal studies that show how oxytocin affects females and males quite differently. [27] [28] [29]

While these aren't the whole picture when it comes to oxytocin in men, there are 3 studies that I find particularly interesting.

In 2022, a study published in *PLOS One* explored how the 'cuddle' hormone impacts stress levels in men versus women. On arrival, 38 couples (40 women and 36 men) completed a questionnaire, had their blood pressure taken, and gave a saliva sample. The saliva was to be later analysed for cortisol – the hormone that would represent their overall stress levels. These initial stress levels were used as a baseline, and the participants then went through an unpleasant experience we will refer to as the *pressure test*. [30]

During the pressure test, participants were instructed to:

1. Keep their hands in ice-cold water for 3 minutes
2. Maintain eye contact with a camera
3. Not speak

If they broke any of these rules, an invigilator in a lab coat made a note. This unpleasant experience was designed to put them under pressure and see what happened to their stress levels. Immediately after the pressure test, their stress levels were taken again, and then at 15 and 25 minutes.

Some of the participants went through the experiment just as I have described, but some had a slightly different experience. Just before the pressure test, some of the participants were instructed to *hug their partner*. This allowed the researchers to test whether the hug protected men against stress, and whether it was as protective for them as the women in the experiment.

Here are some of the findings from the study, starting with women...

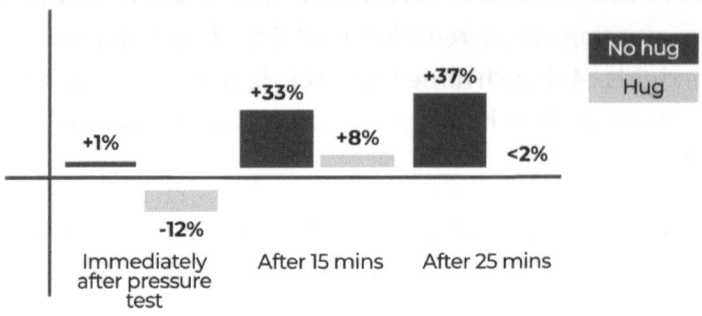

Adapted from R203: G Berretz et al (2022). 'Romantic partner embraces reduce cortisol release after acute stress induction in women but not in men.' PLOS ONE.

In women who did not receive a hug:

- The pressure test increased stress levels by an average of 37%.
- 25 minutes after the pressure test, stress levels had still not returned to baseline.

In women who received a hug:

- The pressure test only increased stress levels by an average of 8%.
- Within 25 minutes, their stress levels had returned to normal.

Not only did the hug significantly reduce the stress response in women, but their stress levels also returned to normal much faster. Now let's look at what happened to the men in this experiment…

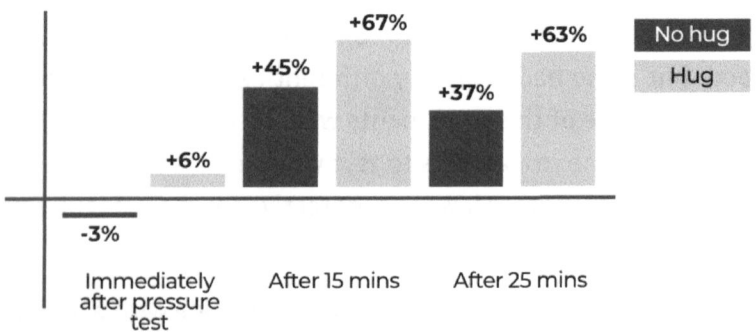

Adapted from R203: G Berretz et al (2022). 'Romantic partner embraces reduce cortisol release after acute stress induction in women but not in men.' PLOS ONE.

In men who did not receive a hug:

- The pressure test increased stress levels by an average of 45%.
- 25 minutes after the pressure test, stress levels were still high, but were starting to reduce.

In men who received a hug:

- The pressure test increased stress levels by an average of 67%!
- By the final saliva test, the most stressed group was men who had received a hug before the pressure test.

The study found a startling difference between women. While adding a hug protected women against stress, it seemed to greatly increase stress levels in men. But the difference was quite played down. The study simply stated:

"No stress-buffering effect could be observed in men." [31]

You have to read the study's average hormone measurements to see that cortisol levels increased more in men who received a hug than men who didn't.

That's 1 study that suggests men and women might need very different forms of support when it comes to dealing with stress. But this experiment used a hug, not actual oxytocin. Let's look at the other 2 studies I found so fascinating in this area. These next 2 studies are both from 2012 and used intranasal oxytocin (oxytocin sprayed into the nose).

One study, published in *Experimental and Clinical Psychopharmacology*, found that intranasal oxytocin reduced stress in some women, but not in men. [32]

The other study, this time published in *Social Cognitive and Affective Neuroscience*, sprayed either oxytocin or a placebo (saline solution) into the noses of arguing partners. They found that, in women, the oxytocin was linked with reduced stress levels. But in men, oxytocin was linked with *increased* stress levels. It made them more co-operative, but it didn't help their cortisol levels. [33]

These studies suggest it's too presumptive to assume that oxytocin has the same stress-buffering effect on males that it has on females. It appears that the relationship between oxytocin and stress levels in men is far more complicated than it is in women!

Before I am misunderstood, I am not suggesting that a single hug or an emotional conversation would ruin an otherwise pleasant day for a man. No, I am simply stating that you can't take studies about oxytocin on women and apply the same conclusions to men.

Remember that one of the studies on relationships earlier in the book warned that:

"Combining men and women in the same models could produce misleading results." [34]

And yet most of the studies on oxytocin seem to be carried out with female participants. In the study we looked at earlier, where children were given different forms of support, only girls were chosen to take part. This was apparently because:

1. Most of the research on oxytocin so far is in females.
2. Boys would be less accepting of physical touch and comforting words due to "social norms".

To me, these are both reasons to *include* boys in the study, not to exclude them! Otherwise we risk building a gender biased view of these hormones. I know that some people don't like discussing biological sex differences in mental health, I think because they worry it will lead to judgement and discrimination. But wouldn't more of an understanding of biological sex differences allow people to better understand one another, and how to support those they love?

The studies suggest that biology may play a big part in why men are less likely to talk about how they feel, and why oxytocin-releasing activities like cuddling, crying, or talking might not work as well for men as they often do for women. That doesn't mean social conditioning has no influence — but it would be wrong to assume the differences are purely down to upbringing when biology clearly plays a role too.

But why does the famous "love" hormone impact men so differently to women? Because oxytocin is not the "love" hormone in males.

Oxytocin has a sibling hormone, called vasopressin. Both oxytocin and vasopressin evolved from an ancient parent hormone called vasotocin. Over time, oxytocin evolved to be the bonding hormone in females and vasopressin became the bonding hormone in males. In animal experiments, blocking oxytocin can prevent female animals from forming an attachment to their partner, whereas **blocking vasopressin has the same effect in males**. [35] [36] [37]

I'm sharing this with you so that next time you hear someone talk about oxytocin being the "love hormone" that "lowers stress", you know they might have a one-sided gender biased view of oxytocin. What's more, I believe that this generalisation completely ignores males and further alienates men from feeling understood.

I regularly work with men who share their lived experience that there is nothing wrong with touching, hugging, crying or talking about how they feel; but *on their own those things don't reduce their stress*. When they do reach out for help, men are often told the same thing: *"You need to talk how you feel."* So when they *are* talking about how they feel and they're not feeling better, they can come to a logical but dangerous conclusion:

"If talking about how I feel is the solution, but it's not working for me, then there must be something wrong with me."

Our message to those men should be that this doesn't mean there is anything wrong with you; in fact, there is a perfectly reasonable scientific explanation for that lived experience.

I believe that talking is vital – for men and women. But for men, talking alone is not the solution, it is simply the first step on the road to finding their solution.

First, men need to know what to talk about, but most importantly, they need to know what to *do* in order to address the issues that are causing them to feel this way.

As Gary put it during one of our coaching calls: *"Talking about how I feel is the price I am prepared to pay to find solutions to my problems. But when I talk about how I feel and there is no solution at the end, I feel I've paid a high price for nothing. When that happens too many times, you learn not to reach out for help. Because it just doesn't help."*

I believe that oxytocin's differing effects in females and males causes 2 big miscommunications. Firstly, it can cause women to believe that men "just need to talk". But it can cause men to believe that talking doesn't work, leading to communication breakdown. And communication breakdown is the main cause of relationship breakdown. But by understanding these biological differences, I think we can become better friends, partners, and allies to those we support.

Protecting the Cave: Strategies

Protecting the Cave is about feeling secure. In this part of the book, we have explored how financial and relationship stability impacts suicide rates in men, and the protective role of security. Understanding the hormonal differences between men and women highlights how we can all support the men we care about by helping them to *address* their issues, not just to *talk about them*.

❏ Express and address underlying issues

Talking about problems is vital, but for men that is only the first step. Next, men need to address the issues that are causing them to feel that way. You can often provide this support by asking 2 simple questions:

1. What's on your mind?
2. What can you do about it?

These 2 questions combine to quickly start an open conversation about practical solutions, and place the focus on him to come up with his own ideas.

It's important to note that the first question is *"What's on your mind?"* rather than *"What's wrong?"* *"How are you feeling today?"* or *"I'm worried about you, is everything OK?"* We'll explore why this wording is important in Part 8: How to Talk to Him.

❏ Review monthly costs

Depending on your relationship to him, it might be appropriate to sit down and review his monthly costs together. When Gary felt overwhelmed by his financial situation, his regular monthly "finance dates" with Emily gave him a sense of clarity and control. Together, they reviewed their spending for the previous month and made decisions about next month's budget. This helped them 'tighten up' where necessary to navigate the current challenge. It also had the added benefit of ensuring they were communicating about the problem and their joint plan to address it.

Once Gary felt in touch with his monthly expenditure, he could calculate how many months' worth of costs he had in the bank, or how long it would take to pay off certain debts once he had an income again. Another advantage of the monthly finance date is that it increases understanding and communication between life partners, business partners, or any 2 people who trust each other enough to share their monthly costs.

❏ Focus on building a monthly surplus

This isn't only appropriate if you are a life or business partner, but to anyone who supports men. Something I have learned from working with men is that men who have debts that they are paying off seem to feel more secure than men who have savings that they are dipping into.

That sense of financial security for men seems to be mainly associated with a sense of whether they are heading in the right or wrong direction. This may be something that you can talk about, or even help with. In some instances, he might require professional financial or legal advice; but in the majority of cases, all that you need to do is to share a calculator and stay focussed on the fundamentals:

Income > costs = financial security
Income < costs = financial insecurity

Once the conversation is in flow, your role is simply to help him to identify ways he can increase his income or reduce his costs. If you are non-judgmental and treat the numbers as a maths problem to be solved, any stigma related to money will melt away and he will usually create a plan himself. If you're not in the position to offer this kind of support, or if the situation is more complicated than you are comfortable with, the next strategy will help.

(I thought it worth adding here that a calculator is part of my standard equipment as a coach, alongside a single £1 coin. The calculator is essential for exploring business and financial issues. I use the coin to help clients who are stuck between two equally appealing—or unappealing—options. The decision is never made by the coin, but I flip it and ask them how they feel about the result. This prompts them either to over-rule the coin or confirm that they are happy with its suggestion. Decision made!)

❏ Team up with money / debt charities (if needed)

In the UK, and throughout many countries in the world, there is a growing number of charities that specialise in helping those struggling with debt, budgeting, or unemployment.

I mentioned the Hope project, because it is an excellent example. But if you don't live close enough to Bristol, UK to use Hope, there are many other charities that recognise the importance of financial security and how it impacts mental health. I signpost to several UK charities on my Resources page, at TheMensCoach.co.uk/resources. Their support is free.

❏ Spend quality time with partner (if relevant)

I find that the conversation around oxytocin impacting females and males in different ways is useful for helping men (including me) realise the importance of quality time. Unfortunately, a common regret of many men is that they "didn't spend enough quality time" with their partner, and didn't realise until it was "too late". Ironically, this is often because they were showing their dedication in another way - being a provider.

You may be in a position to encourage him to have quality time with his partner. If you are his partner, many other partners have fed back to me that just sitting down together and talking about the differences of oxytocin has significantly improved their relationship, their understanding of one another, and their (potentially) differing needs. Men are used to being told that we don't talk about how we feel because of the way we were raised, so to hear a hormonal explanation for this phenomenon can help men to feel more understood and less inclined to give up when talking alone isn't the solution.

Ultimately, our aim here is to support men to address the financial and relationship issues that can lead to insecurity. It requires courage and directness but it can quickly restore his sense of security. These 5 strategies do that by encouraging men to tackle the issues head on.

ENDNOTES

1. R819: L Lu et al. (2020). "Gender difference in suicidal ideation and related factors among rural elderly: a cross-sectional study in Shandong, China." Annals of General Psychiatry.
2. R672: National Confidential Inquiry into Suicide and Safety in Mental Health (2021). "Suicide by middle-aged men." University of Manchester.
3. R158: Samaritans (2012). "Men, Suicide and Society: Why disadvantaged men in midlife die by suicide." samaritans.org.
4. R894: Office for National Statistics (2023). "Sociodemographic inequalities in suicides in England and Wales: 2011 to 2021." ons.gov.uk.
5. R1513: Equimundo (2025). State of American Men 2025. equimundo.org.
6. R1263: N Meda et al. (2021). "The impact of macroeconomic factors on suicide in 175 countries over 27 years." Suicide and Life-Threatening Behavior.
7. R686: Second Step (2023). "Hope Project." second-step.co.uk.
8. R141: J Jackson et al. (2022). "Preventing male suicide through a psychosocial intervention that provides psychological support and tackles financial difficulties: a mixed method evaluation." BMC Psychiatry.
9. R718: S Watts et al. (2013). "CBT for depression: a pilot RCT comparing mobile phone vs. computer." BMC Psychiatry. This is a good example study to use as a comparison, as it also used the PHQ-9 to measure depression but in an 80% female group.
10. R430: A Skinner et al. (2023). "Unemployment and underemployment are causes of suicide." Science Advances.
11. R1188: A Kposowa (2000). "Marital status and suicide in the National Longitudinal Mortality Study." Journal of Epidemiology & Community Health.
12. R1416: C Cantor & P Slater (1995). "Marital breakdown, parenthood, and suicide." Journal of Family Studies.

13 R160: M J Player et al. (2012). "Sociological autopsy: An integrated approach to the study of suicide in men." Social Science & Medicine.
14 R894: Office for National Statistics (2023). "Sociodemographic inequalities in suicides in England and Wales: 2011 to 2021." ons.gov.uk.
15 R579: A S Smith et al. (2017). "Local oxytocin tempers anxiety by activating GABA-A receptors in the hypothalamic paraventricular nucleus." Psychoneuroendocrinology.
16 R1417: T Insel et al. (1998). "Oxytocin, vasopressin, and the neuroendocrine basis of pair bond formation." Advances in Experimental Medicine and Biology.
17 R1498: Stockholm University (2025). "Oxytocin – The key to social bonds?" su.se/department-of-psychology/news
18 R896: C Crockford et al. (2013). "Urinary oxytocin and social bonding in related and unrelated wild chimpanzees." Proceedings of the Royal Society B: Biological Sciences.
19 R1418: N Brondino et al. (2017). "Something to talk about: Gossip increases oxytocin levels in a near real-life situation." Psychoneuroendocrinology.
20 R1419: C Raypole (2020). "12 ways to boost oxytocin." HealthLine.com.
21 R208: L J Seltzer (2012). "Instant messages vs. speech: hormones and why we still need to hear each other." Evolution and Human Behavior.
22 R1045: S Moffatt et al (1996). "Salivary testosterone concentrations in left-handers: An association with cerebral language lateralization." Neuropsychologia.
23 R1047: J Pennebaker et al (2022). "Testosterone as a Social Inhibitor: Two Case Studies of the Effect of Testosterone Treatment on Language." Journal of Psychopathology and Clinical Science.
24 R1452: J Doom et al (2016). "Social stress buffering by friends in childhood and adolescence: Effects on HPA and oxytocin activity." Social Neuroscience.
25 R1236: D Marazziti et al (2019). "Sex-Related Differences in Plasma Oxytocin Levels in Humans." Clinical Practice & Epidemiology in Mental Health.
26 R222: A Lane et al (2012). "Oxytocin increases willingness to socially share one's emotions." International Journal of Psychology.
27 R1420: J Rilling et al. (2013). "Sex differences in the neural and behavioral response to intranasal oxytocin and vasopressin during human social interaction." Psychoneuroendocrinology.
28 R205: S Gao et al. (2016). "Oxytocin, the peptide that bonds the sexes also divides them." Proceedings of the National Academy of Sciences. This article title inspired the names of the two oxytocin chapters in this book: "The hormone that bonds us" and "The hormone that divides us."
29 R1501: P Duarte-Guterman et al. (2020). "Oxytocin has sex-specific effects on social behaviour and hypothalamic oxytocin immunoreactive cells but not hippocampal neurogenesis in adult rats." Hormones and Behaviour.
30 R203: G Berretz et al. (2022). "Romantic partner embraces reduce cortisol release after acute stress induction in women but not in men." PLOS One.
31 R203: G Berretz et al. (2022).

32 R155: C Cardoso et al. (2012). "Coping style moderates the effect of intranasal oxytocin on the mood response to interpersonal stress." Experimental and Clinical Psychopharmacology.
33 R630: B Ditzen et al. (2013). "Sex-specific effects of intranasal oxytocin on autonomic nervous system and emotional responses to couple conflict." Social Cognitive and Affective Neuroscience.
34 R1188: A Kposowa (2000). "Marital status and suicide in the National Longitudinal Mortality Study." Journal of Epidemiology & Community Health.
35 R1493: H Caldwell et al. (2017). "Oxytocin and vasopressin: Powerful regulators of social behavior." The Neuroscientist.
36 R358: C S Carter et al. (2019). "The monogamy paradox: What do love and sex have to do with it?" Frontiers in Ecology and Evolution.
37 R1417: T Insel et al. (1998). "Oxytocin, vasopressin, and the neuroendocrine basis of pair bond formation." Advances in Experimental Medicine and Biology.

PART 5

HAVING ADVENTURES

"Life is either a daring adventure or nothing at all"
— Helen Keller

	Having Adventures
Signs of stress	- Life *flying by* - Lack of motivation or discipline - Working all the time - Procrastination - Distractions / cravings (eg: porn, alcohol, social media etc.)

Ryan's story

In November 2018, I was in the sea off the coast of Brazil. And I was fighting for my life.

This was before I heard about Brad, and before I met my wife Emma. I was on holiday with some friends and I was supposed to be kitesurfing.

Kitesurfing is a water sport where you attach yourself by harness to a large, inflatable kite and ride what looks like a surfboard on the sea. It feels like you are flying across the water, and I loved it. But the reason I say "supposed to be kitesurfing" is that things took a very bad turn, very quickly.

My friends and I had been on a 10k "downwinder" – that's a journey along the coast, in the same direction of the wind, so you can cover distances quicker and enjoy the scenery. Being the least experienced, they waited as long as they could for me, but then made progress at their own speed. I don't blame them; it was their holiday too. My friend Helena stayed relatively close to me to ensure I was never kiting alone. She was on her own kite and her own board. But the conditions meant that she couldn't get close enough to me to warn me about what was going on. By the time I realised what was happening, it was too late.

I was way out from the shore and hadn't read the sea – or the situation – at all. While the water had been flat when we set out, I was now riding over what I can only describe as large rolling *hills* of water. These hills were metres high, and yet the wind had grown weaker and weaker. I was working my kite harder and harder just to generate enough pull to keep me standing on my board. Then, the wind died. My kite stalled and fluttered down to the sea where it landed out of my sight – behind one of the large hills of water. Thud. I tried for several minutes to launch the kite again, but with no wind, I was wasting what little time I had left to save myself.[1]

I couldn't see the land or my friend Helena. I knew she was either in the same situation, or she had headed to land to get help. Most of the time, I couldn't even see my kite. It was a struggle just keeping my head above the water, as the large hills of water passed straight over me, as if I wasn't there. The reality of the situation began to dawn on me.

I was alone. Wearing no life jacket. In a sea with no lifeguard. Off a coast that had no phone signal. Miles away from the nearest town.

In situations like this, the safest thing to do is to get onto your kite. After all, it is a large, brightly coloured inflatable. Even if you can't ride it ashore, at least it floats and will be easier to spot if you are washed out to sea, compared to a head bobbing amongst waves. If anyone was even looking for me... But they weren't.

However, you can't just swim to your kite. I was connected to the kite by several long, strong lines – each about 60 feet – that act like cables. If I was to swim toward the kite, the lines would go slack and sink. And if the lines were to snag on something underwater, the kite's buoyancy pulling up could easily drag me down. To reach the kite safely, I had to wind up the lines while staying afloat – a manoeuvre kiters call a '*deep water pack down.*' It's extremely difficult. And I just couldn't do it.

I had finally wound in about half the length of the cables, when the kite broke free from the "water hills" and into steep, aggressive walls of waves, heading at speed for the beach. The cables – along with all my hard work – were ripped from my hands as the kite tore away from me.

It was at this point that I realised I had also made another big mistake. Before I took to the water, I had connected the '*second stage safety*' – that's the final cable that connected me to the kite – to the back of my harness. This meant that if the kite was deactivated (which it was), and I tried to wind it in (which I did), and it broke away from me (which it had), the kite would drag me along backwards.

And so, as my kite was seized by a wave, the cables torn from my hands, I was spun around, pulled under the water, and dragged behind the kite, backwards and upside down.

Water burned and pushed its way up my nose and into my throat. I wanted to scream, but an instinct took over that kept my mouth closed tight. I tried to look around, but there was nothing to see. I was able to use 1 hand to reach around my back and hold the taut cable that was pulling me through, and under, the water.

I knew that it would be dangerous to disconnect from the kite. I didn't know whether the tide was coming in or going out. If it was going out, I would be taken out with it, and waste the last of my energy fighting it. But even if the tide was coming in, I didn't know what kind of land I would swim into. It could be a vertical cliff face with no escape.

But I also knew that if I didn't disconnect from the kite, I would drown in the next 60 seconds. I was being pulled into a sea of total darkness, not knowing which way to turn. And all I could feel was regret.

Only, it wasn't the regret that you might expect. I didn't regret the trip to Brazil, or my decision to join my friends on the downwinder. I didn't regret the fact that our hire shop didn't stock life jackets. I didn't regret the fact that I hadn't realised the rolling hills and the dying wind were signals that I should return to the shore. I didn't regret that I had missed Helena's warning signals. I didn't regret the time I spent trying to relaunch my kite, or having the cable stupidly attached to my back, or the water forcing its way into my throat. I regretted the way I had lived my adult life up until that day.

You see, for the previous 5 years, my life had revolved around alcohol. I would repeatedly drink too much and regret it the next day. And then I'd do the exact same thing the following evening. It was as if, the more I regretted it, the more I needed to do it again. Every occasion was an excuse to drink alcohol. When I had a good day, I would drink to celebrate. When I had a bad day, I would drink to escape my problems. I would drink with friends, at parties, and alone on my sofa. In the year leading up to Brazil, I had probably drunk alcohol every day. Half a litre of vodka, at home, alone on a Tuesday night was normal for me. I would often fall asleep on my sofa, in my clothes, having had no dinner, without even brushing my teeth.

When I drank at parties, I was not a nice person. I would be loud, pushy, and rude. I didn't want to be, but once I started drinking, I couldn't help it. I became impulsive. I would say stupid things and make stupid decisions. Everyone knew me as a "party guy". Everyone knew I was up for going clubbing every day, regardless of the consequences. When they found out that I had died in Brazil, never recovered from the sea, I knew exactly what people would say:

"Well, I'm not surprised. I bet he was drunk at the time."

I would be remembered by many as rude, drunk, and impulsive. I would be remembered for the parties I crashed, the barbeques I ruined, and the nightclubs I threw up in. I knew that if I died here in the sea, that's the legacy I would leave. I imagined my mum having to get a passport to fly to Brazil to see the sea that I had been lost in.

And that's when I realised that I was about to do it. I was about to detach myself from the kite, detach myself from the only thing that floated in this entire sea and take my chances in the waves. I knew that the waves, the tide, or the shore could kill me. But I knew I had to try. I could not be remembered like this.

I squeezed the safety release with my right thumb. The cable tore away through the water, under fierce pressure. The kite was gone. It was all on me now. I had to get to the beach.

My head rose out of the water and I opened my mouth to breathe again, just in time to swallow a wave that rode straight over me. I tumbled in the darkness again, desperate to get the water out of my nose and air into my lungs. Finally, my head broke free from the water and I snatched a gasp of air before another wave went over my head.

Over the following few minutes, I got into a routine of catching a breath before the next wave forced me under again. And then I got my bearings and began swimming in the same general direction as the waves. *"Surely,"* I thought... *"Surely the waves are heading towards the beach?"* I had no way of knowing. All I could see were the sea, the sky and the waves that connected them.

I had never swum like this before. Every cell in my body was exploding with energy and purpose. Every inch of every finger and limb heaved and kicked the water. Every part of my body answered the call of the shore, though I had no idea if it was anywhere near. As each wave hit me, I fought harder. Tears ran down my cheeks, sea water flowed from my nose and over my chin as I punched, and kicked, and tore through the water. *"Please..."* I thought. *"Please let the tide be coming in..."*

As I forced my way through the water, there was a moment where I looked ahead and I saw a wall of waves: 2 metres high and as wide as the horizon, heading calmly along with all the force of nature. The setting sun danced in the reflection on their backs. I remember thinking that this was the most beautiful final thing to see, and I was so lucky to have this last moment, alone. Then, it happened.

Trees over the tops of the waves! I couldn't believe it.

I just hoped they wouldn't be sitting on top of a vertical cliff face that was waiting for me. A vertical cliff face with no way of escape. I desperately hoped that those trees were on a beach. And then…

Yellow sand.

I emerged from the water, dripping, coughing, and laughing. Helena – who had been running along the beach looking for me – ran towards me. We embraced. *"Are you OK?"* she shouted.

"I have never felt better," I replied. My kite lay ripped and tangled on the beach next to me. We had made it.

I would love to tell you that I never drank any alcohol since, but it wasn't like that. Although I now had a reason to give up drinking, I wasn't ready to actually do it.

For another 5 weeks, I continued drinking alcohol every night. By New Year's Eve 2018, I knew it was now or never. But the idea of not drinking alcohol was the single most frightening idea I could imagine. I had no idea who I was without it.

The only way I could possibly be happy about it was to tell myself, *"If I can do this, I can do absolutely anything."* I told my friends and my partner at the time (she was very supportive) that I was going to be sober for the next 16 months until my 30th birthday party.

That evening, as the nightclub erupted with noise and everyone counted down to midnight, I inhaled 2 large double vodkas in cheap imitation cola. I drank them like water. They were all I had left.

What happened next? The first 21 days were hard. Very hard. But after that, things became easier. After a few months, not only did I feel better for not drinking, but other things became easier too. With each month of sobriety, my discipline grew. So did my motivation and my focus.

I didn't understand it at the time, but the months and years that followed without drinking were undoing the damage that alcohol had caused to the parts of my brain that are needed for motivation, discipline and for decision-making. With my knowledge now, I understand why.

While I was able to stop drinking alcohol on my own, some people can have a physical dependence on alcohol that could make it dangerous – or even fatal – to stop suddenly. DrinkAware.co.uk contains tools to help people understand whether they might be dependent on alcohol, and how to safely cut down or stop.

I had to share my story at this point in the book. Yes, I have a lot of experience helping men to understand the other Dimensions of The ALPHA Framework. But **Having Adventures** is the Dimension that personally impacted me the most. I know what it's like to spend all working day thinking about the alcohol you will have when you get home. And I know what it does to every other part of your life, and to every other thought. I also now understand enough of the science to explain what was happening in my brain with every sip, and with every drink.

I understand now why my decision to stop drinking alcohol had such a profound impact on so many areas of my life. My use of alcohol had been both a symptom of, and partly the cause of, an even bigger problem: dopamine dysregulation.

The H in ALPHA stands for **Having Adventures**. It's about the things men need to do for their sense of motivation and discipline.

Having Adventures: The science

Dopamine: The molecule of motivation

Have you ever been asked what you did yesterday, and not been able to remember? Or come home from work and realised that you have no memory of the day? Come to think of it, can you remember any details from your last drive to work?

I'm not talking about memory loss here. I'm talking about all the drives to work, repetitive tasks, and familiar routines that just seem to blur into one. If you can't remember them either, don't worry – it doesn't mean that there is anything wrong with your brain.

But isn't it curious that there are some things that happened to you 10 years, 20 years, or 40 years ago that you can remember as if they were yesterday. And yet half the things you did today you have already forgotten? Why are some memories etched into our mind forever, while some are never even taken in?

It's to do with the way your brain works.

Despite only making up about 2% of your weight, your brain uses over 20% of your energy. Your brain is so energy costly that we have developed ways to keep the energy bill down. [2]

When you are doing something repetitive, routine, or familiar, your brain switches into autopilot. Formally called *"procedural memory"*, autopilot allows your brain to use less energy and stops you from recording new memories. This way, you save energy and avoid stockpiling hours of memories of washing the dishes, driving to work, and filling in spreadsheets. [3] [4]

The end result is that you can complete entire car journeys, weeks at work, or even months of your life without creating any new memories. This is good news for your brain, but bad news for your perception of time.

It seems to me that as you grow older, you become more competent and settle into a familiar routine in a familiar environment. This means you spend more time in autopilot mode.

The more time you spend in autopilot mode: the fewer memories you create.

The fewer memories you create: the faster your life seems to pass you by.

And so, the older you become: the faster time seems to pass by.

So how do you break out of this trap?

You introduce some variety into your life. You get out of your comfort zone. Because when you do *new* things, meet *new* people, or learn something *new*, your brain releases a chemical messenger called dopamine. [5]

Dopamine has many functions in your body, but in this book, we're interested in the role it plays within the brain.

When dopamine is released in the brain, it fires up pathways that are associated with **motivation** and **movement**. So you feel compelled to act. But the release of dopamine also informs the memory centres in your brain that what's happening is important, causing **new memories** to be created. In this way, dopamine "tags" events in your life, which is why you remember the new places, new people, and the new experiences, while all the repetitive things you do just blur into one. [6]

If you've ever noticed that 7 days of holiday create lifelong memories, but you can't remember any of your last 462 drives to work, you've already experienced this. [7] In fact, we have a word for things that are different enough to cause us to remember them: "memorable".

As the molecule of motivation, dopamine is thought to have evolved to encourage mammals to explore new places and forage for food. It drives mammals out of their safe hiding places and into the big, dangerous world in search of new and exciting things. By boosting or blocking dopamine in monkeys, scientists can make them more or less interested in new things. [8] [9]

Dopamine is a powerful teacher that makes mammals repeat rewarding behaviour and avoid unrewarding activities. When we try to do things that our brain does not associate with reward (like completing a tax return), dopamine is low, which inhibits movement (starting the tax return). I believe that this is where procrastination comes from. It's a protective mechanism designed to stop us from doing things that our brain thinks will be unrewarding.

In prehistoric times, where success depended upon finding food and preserving energy, this simple system was probably ideal. But this is a problem for us today, where success in our modern and complex society often requires us to be able to ignore our short-term impulses and act in line with our long-term goals.

Anyway, what has all this got to do with male mental health?

I regularly work with men who share that their "*life is flying by*", or that they've "*lost motivation*", and it's a sign to me that they need to take a break from the day-to-day routine. But recognising when to take a break is something that some men are extremely bad at.

One man I worked with – Jaden, you'll meet him in part 6 – was working as a security manager in London, but he had previously been a soldier. When I talked to him about dopamine and how I believe this means we need to take regular breaks from our routine to recharge our motivation, he stood up from his seat! As we were having a Zoom call at the time, this meant I couldn't see his face any more, just his chest and waist. But I could hear him…

"Do you realise what this *means*, brother?!" he boomed. "When I was stateside [working in the US], we used to get 35 days of annual leave per year. If you didn't use them, you could carry them forward. But you could only carry forward 70 days, and you lost all the rest. For my squad, it was a badge of honour to always carry forward those 70 days and lose the rest. It was part of what we saw as being a team player. Taking time off was like letting the others down. When I left the military and started working in security, I carried on doing the exact same thing. I haven't taken a break in years! No wonder my life is flying by and I'm lacking motivation… *I need a break!*"

I asked him what he was going to do about it.

"I know exactly what to do," he said. He sat down again, and opened both hands as if he was about to catch something. Something had just clicked into place. "When I leave this coaching call, I'm going to go to my partner and hand her my diary. I'm going to tell her: '*I have 25 days of annual leave that I need to take before the end of year. I would love to spend that time with you.*' Man, I bet my time off will be booked before I know it. She is always telling me I work too much, and that we need to go away. And I always say I can't go away, I'm too busy. I've even cancelled short weekend breaks at the last minute because something came up! No wonder I am lacking motivation. I need to take my adventures as seriously as I take my work!"

Jaden and his partner did start using the holiday he had acquired. At first, he found it very hard to "switch off". But like anything else, it became easier with more practice. They found they didn't need to spend large amounts of money either; small, local adventures were enough to recharge his motivation and create positive new memories.

However, while a steady supply of dopamine from life adventures is essential for our motivation and enjoyment of life, there are certain substances, technologies, and even situations that can hijack our motivation system. This turns dopamine from the molecule of motivation into the chemical of craving.

Unfortunately, this happens every day. To all of us. Let me explain...

Dopamine: The chemical of craving

Some substances cause so much dopamine to be released – and so quickly (often referred to as a "spike") – that normal dopamine regulation is disrupted.

To understand how this impacts you, I am going to talk you through what would happen in your brain if you used a dangerous stimulant like cocaine. [10]

Within microseconds, your brain goes into overdrive, firing dopamine through pathways associated with motivation and movement. You feel euphoric, driven, and restless. You feel the need to move. Even when you try to stand still, your jaw grinds and your head nods. When you sit down, your feet tap and your fingers drum on the table.

The sudden rush of dopamine temporarily disrupts circuits in your brain associated with decision-making, making you impulsive. You say things you normally wouldn't. You do things you will come to regret later. With sound decision-making impaired, taking *more cocaine* seems like a great idea. We can call this the "*binge* stage".

But the binge cannot last forever. Eventually you stop using the cocaine (probably because you've run out). Those motivation and movement circuits that were previously so active are now very quiet.

Your brain panics. You enter *withdrawal*.

Compared to the motivated state you were in, this lack of dopamine feels terrible. You now have to deal with the consequences of the binge. You can't sleep, and you can't take back the things you said or the things you did that were so out of character for you. Your amygdala (the part of your brain that responds to perceived danger) is also suffering, triggering your brain to release stress hormones. So now you feel anxious and stressed. This is what we could call the *regret* stage. You might find yourself thinking, *"I wish I'd never used this drug."*

Despite how terrible the withdrawal feels, dopamine levels and sensitivity will return to normal. Your brain just needs time. But there is another stage in this vicious cycle. You might think that, having experienced the high of the binge and the low of the regret, you would be less likely to use this drug again. But the opposite is true.

During the binge, your brain was firing dopamine into centres linked to decision-making (the prefrontal cortex) and habit formation (the striatum). Your brain now associates the sights, smells, and situations that led to the binge with reward. This starts to shape future decision-making and lays the foundations of a new habit. The same motivation system that once helped our ancestors find food is now hunting for cues related to cocaine. [11] [12]

If you do use the drug again, you'll find that your brain has desensitised, trying to prevent overstimulation. This means that, next time, you will need more cocaine to feel the same high (we touched on something similar when it comes to alcohol tolerance). It also means that you will find other things less rewarding too. [13] [14]

I want to stop for a moment and recognise that you might not have liked me talking so explicitly about cocaine. Cocaine is illegal (in many countries). But cocaine isn't the only thing that interacts with our dopamine levels, impacting our motivation, decision-making, and habits. While they may not be as dangerous or powerful as cocaine, there are other substances that alter the way you think in quite a similar way. But unlike cocaine, some of these are legal and socially acceptable – and even **in the food we give to children**.

Things that "spike" dopamine

Many studies have shown that all addictive drugs "spike" dopamine in the brain. Stimulants like amphetamines (which include "speed") directly boost dopamine release, particularly in the brain's reward areas. The more dopamine they cause to be released (or the more they block the brain's ability to re-absorb the dopamine that is released), the more pleasurable — and addictive — the experience tends to be. [15]

Methylphenidate (a stimulant often prescribed to treat ADHD under brand names Ritalin, Concerta, and others) is designed by drug manufacturers to be as slow-releasing as possible, to try to smooth out the "spike" and withdrawal. But there can still be a withdrawal when it wears off. Some of my clients who have used methylphenidate have found that they feel irritable and lethargic when it wears off, promoting them to use more. Like any medication, this has to be weighed against the reduced symptoms and improved quality of life.

Some addictive drugs indirectly cause dopamine spikes. Opioids like morphine, codeine, and fentanyl act on opiate receptors, while cannabis acts on cannabinoid receptors. Both opiate and cannabinoid receptors can trigger a chain reaction in the brain that releases dopamine. Interestingly, these are the same receptors activated during exercise, producing what's often called the 'runner's high'. [16] [17]

And then there are "*legal highs*". In the lead-up to 2016, the UK Government realised that new street drugs were being introduced faster than the law could ban them. As a result, the UK Government created a new law (Psychoactive Substances Act 2016) to ban any drugs which work "*by stimulating or depressing the person's central nervous system, [affecting] the person's mental functioning or emotional state.*" [18]

However, a list of exempted substances had to be added, to prevent the law from banning the sale of **alcohol**, **cigarettes**, **vaping**, **coffee** and **energy drinks!** These are all products that spike our dopamine levels, causing a withdrawal and potential addiction, but are socially acceptable and even generate tax revenue for governments around the world.

The Psychoactive Substances Act also had to **make an exception for food**. While you may have been aware of the effects drugs and alcohol can have on our central nervous system, you may be surprised to hear there are many ways that **foods can impact our dopamine levels.**

Foods that raise our blood sugar quickly — like white bread, pastries, rice, and breakfast cereal — often leaving us feeling hungry again soon after. These "highs" and "lows" activate our dopamine system, causing food cravings, overeating and potential addiction. [19] [20]

Unfortunately, dietary advice tends to focus on eating less, rather than eating less addictive food. In fact, many of the foods that cause these cravings are often marketed as healthy, on the basis that they are "low in fat" or lower total cholesterol (see Part 3: Looking After Body & Mind as a reminder as to why low total cholesterol is not always a good thing, especially for men over the age of 35!).

When I deliver workshops on dopamine, I'm often asked whether it's possible to be "addicted" to bread or cheese. Interestingly, gluten (found in bread, bagels, and pastries) and casein (found in dairy) break down into substances called *exorphins*, which can activate opiate receptors in the gut. We don't yet have human research showing whether exorphins can cause physical dependence — but we do know that drugs which act on the same opiate receptors (such as Loperamide, sold as Imodium) can cause physical dependence if used long-term. In those cases, withdrawal can include anxiety, irritability, and low mood. [21] [22] [23] [24]

Many ultra-processed foods combine bread with dairy - think of cheeseburgers, pizza or 'loaded' fries. If the exorphines from bread and dairy have a similar effect to drugs which activate the same receptors, this could explain another reason why ultra-processed foods can be hard to stop eating.

Just to be clear, I'm not saying ultra-processed food is as dangerous as cocaine or speed. Let's keep things in perspective here. What I am saying is that if you've ever promised yourself you'd stop eating this kind of thing — and then found yourself reaching for it anyway — you're not lazy or weak.

You're up against substances that may be hijacking your biology in multiple ways.

Bright screens are another thing that probably interfere with our dopamine system. In one animal study, rats were exposed to lights of different intensities, and the greatest dopamine activity occurred at around 32 lux (a measure of how much brightness our eyes actually receive). By contrast, an iPhone 16 probably delivers something like 1,400 lux to your eyes. There aren't yet human studies confirming whether our dopamine circuits respond to light in the same way as other animals, but given how much time we spend looking at screens, I think those studies are seriously overdue. (Check the footnote if you're curious how I estimated the lux of an iPhone screen.) [25] [26] [27]

As I alluded to earlier, it's thought that dopamine evolved to motivate mammals to forage for food, particularly fruit. As a result, our brain's reward system seems to be activated by bright, contrasting colours (think of ripe fruit against green leaves) and round red shapes, like berries. Whether deliberately designed or accidentally achieved, modern smartphones contain this mix of colour and round red circles that are called notifications. In a 2023 experiment published in *Computers in Human Behavior Reports*, participants went from using their phones in full colour, to using them in black and white mode all day. This reduced screen time, phone addiction, and made users happier about their relationship with their phone – after just 24 hours. This simple change blocks one of the ways that your smartphone probably interacts with your brain. [28]

At the time of publishing, you can put an iPhone into black and white using "Greyscale". Android is a little trickier. You have to turn on "Bedtime Mode" which will also activate "Do Not Disturb". Of course, you can simply then turn Do Not Disturb off. I'll talk you through this in more detail in the Strategies part of this section.

And then there are certain situations that can hijack your dopamine system. Yes, situations. To understand why they do this, you need to understand a concept we are going to call **variable reward**. [29]

Simply put, variable reward is when you do something predictable, but the reward is unpredictable. When you get a reward that you couldn't predict, it releases more dopamine than a predictable one.

This probably traces back to dopamine's role in encouraging mammals to forage for food. They walk to the bush that sometimes contains berries [predictable action], and they may or may not find berries [unpredictable reward]. But in the modern world, this same mechanism can lead to unwanted cravings and compulsive behaviour.

Take gambling, for example. You roll a dice [predictable action] and you *might* win by rolling a high number [unpredictable reward]. Or you pull the arm of a slot machine [predictable action] and you *might* win the jackpot [unpredictable reward]. Of course, you're far more likely to lose your money.

Men I have worked with who were struggling with gambling addiction often shared stories of an "*early win*" that they believe got them hooked. And have you ever noticed how slot machines (also called fruit machines) are often covered in images of juicy red cherries that signal a win? It's as if we're back to foraging for fruit again…

Variable reward has been found to create habits that are extremely hard to quit. Gambling, gaming, and shopping all involve repetitive actions and unpredictable rewards. This tricks our brains into thinking that we are foraging for something valuable. In reality, we are just consuming a product, often designed to be addictive in the first place. But what happens when the addictiveness of variable reward is combined with the addictiveness of a bright screen?

In 2002, Google News was one of the first websites to use an algorithm to collate different news headlines and articles. It wasn't sophisticated enough to tailor the articles to each individual reader, but that didn't matter at the time. Each time you visited, the headlines were different – new stories added, old ones moved down, and breaking news could appear at any time. This unpredictability made checking Google News exciting, like opening a present. People began to refresh their browser to see whether anything new had appeared. (Funnily enough, the word *"news"* comes from Middle-English *newes*, which was the plural of "new". It literally means "new things". No wonder it stimulates dopamine!)

In 2006, Facebook took this even further when they added a page with a personalised algorithm that gave you tailored updates on your friends without visiting their profiles. They called it the News Feed.

The News Feed allowed you to scroll down [predictable action] and get updates on what your friends were up to [unpredictable reward]. Newsfeeds have since become a staple of social media, with sites like YouTube, Instagram, and TikTok delivering highly personalised short video content which has the power to keep you "doomscrolling" for hours. In 2025, the UK's 10 most visited websites all integrate some form of variable reward, encouraging you to forage for new content each time you visit. [30]

The end result is we can often find ourselves endlessly scrolling through social media, constantly checking our phone, or repeatedly reading our emails, compulsively seeking a reward.

If you think that this is accidental, rather than intentional, you just need to read some blogs on app design. You'll see that app designers go to great efforts to ensure that their products create repetitive behaviours – integrating newsfeeds, notifications, and "like" counters. Once one app finds a way to be more addictive, the others soon follow. In the words of Edward Tufte of Yale University: *"There are only two industries that call their customers 'users': illegal drugs and software."* [31]

I'm not sharing this in order to make app designers seem like bad people, or suggesting that we don't benefit enormously from modern technology. My aim is only to give some insight on why we might find ourselves stuck for hours on certain apps. Especially the ones that make us scroll, check notifications, or read messages.

What I've shared with you so far in this section affects people of all genders. But here is something that seems particularly relevant to the men we care about…

Before 2007, only around 2–5% of men under the age of 40 were thought to have erectile dysfunction (ED). By 2011, the figure had risen to 45%, according to 1 review study. That includes males aged between 16 and 21. What could have possibly caused such a steep increase in ED? [32]

In 2007, adult websites began to resemble their own kind of news feed — offering endless scrolling of videos, personalised content, and fast-loading clips on a bright screen. While pornography has been around for hundreds of years in different forms, this new combination of nudity, novelty, and easy escalation became a highly stimulating and addictive experience, especially for males.

One brain scan study involved 31 men—17 regular cocaine users and 14 non-users—who watched videos related to cocaine use, pornography, and nature scenes. When the non-users watched porn, their brain's reward centers were activated in a similar way to how the cocaine users' brains responded when watching cocaine-related videos. [33]

In fact, this combination is so stimulating for the male brain, that it seems to desensitise motivation circuits, causing poor quality erections and lack of interest in sex with a regular partner. [34]

And being young doesn't seem to offer protection against this:

"A 2016 study [...] assessed sexual problems in adolescents (16–21 years) [...]. For males, persistent problems were low sexual satisfaction (47.9%), low desire (46.2%), and problems in erectile function (45.3%). The researchers noted that over time rates of sexual problems declined for females, but not for males." [35]

In 2017, researcher Samuel Perry analysed data from the Portrait of American Life Study ("PALS" for short). As part of PALS, 1,000 people completed a detailed questionnaire in 2006 about their life, and then again in 2012.

Perry found that the single best predictor of relationship quality in married couples in 2012 was relationship quality in 2006. That probably isn't a surprise: if you're having a good relationship now, it's more likely to be good in 6 years time. But Perry found that the second-best predictor of relationship quality — out of hundreds of data points — was the amount of porn that the male partner watched. [36]

In men, watching porn "*a few times a month*" or more in 2006 strongly predicted worse relationship quality in 2012 (I would suggest here that "*a few times a month*" is a very small amount of porn, compared to many men). The more porn men watched, the more their relationship quality declined over the following 6 years. The only answer to the question "*How often do you watch porn?*" that predicted better than average relationship quality in 6 years' time was "*Never*".

(Conversely, in women, more porn use was associated with an improvement in relationship quality over the study period.)

But here's where it gets really interesting. A year later, Perry looked at the same data but from another angle: relationship *stability*. Remember that relationships are extremely protective for men, and separation is associated with significant increased risk of suicide.

In both females and males, "*never*" watching porn was associated with a low risk of separation over the following 6 years. Watching porn "*a few times a month*" was associated with a 3× increased risk of relationship breakdown over the study period. But once partners are watching porn more than "*a few times a month*", the risk of splitting up actually **declines with more porn use.** [37]

Combining the same data used in these 2 studies, it appears that:

- When men "*never*" watch porn, relationship quality increases over time, and there is a low risk of separation.
- When men watch porn "*a few times a month*", relationship quality tends to worsen and there is a 3× increased risk of separation.
- When men watch porn most days, relationship quality strongly deteriorates over time, but they seem to lose the motivation to fix it or to end the relationship (my conclusion).

It looks like internet porn poses a significant risk to males – being so available, addictive, and damaging. Despite this, research suggests that mental health support is not equipped to help men with this issue at all:

"Because Internet pornography-related sexual difficulties are not yet specifically encompassed in an official diagnosis, healthcare providers do not routinely screen for them, leaving patients vulnerable." [38]

Instead, many men may be treated with counselling for "performance anxiety" or given prescription medications to help with their erections, when all they need is time without porn for their brain to normalise.

This is disappointing, because so often I see that just knowing about the damage porn causes to the male brain and erection quality is enough to encourage most men and boys to decide to take a break from it.

So, to summarise, some of the things that can spike dopamine include:

- Stimulants like cocaine, amphetamines, methylphenidate
- Opiates like morphine, codeine, fentanyl
- Cannabinoids like cannabis (marijuana)
- Legal highs like alcohol, nicotine, and caffeine
- Food that includes sugar, starch, gluten, dairy
- Bright screens, like the kind on phones, tablets, TVs
- Variable reward: gambling, gaming, shopping
- Scrolling: newsfeeds, social media, message inboxes
- Internet porn

If you're wondering why I am so interested in things that we can become addicted to, it's because they seem to have a much greater effect on our mental health than many people think...

How dopamine dysregulation impacts motivation and discipline

In a study published in 2020 in *Addiction Science & Clinical Practice*, researchers compared health records from 2,674 people who died by suicide with 267,400 similar people who were still alive, across 8 US healthcare systems over 13 years. The study looked at whether addictions to substances like tobacco, alcohol, and drugs increase the risk of dying by suicide in everyday men and women across the US. [39]

The research found that every type of addiction studied – drugs, alcohol, and even smoking tobacco – was linked to a higher risk of suicide, even after considering other factors like age and socioeconomic status.

People addicted to tobacco were about twice as likely to die by suicide, while those addicted to tobacco, alcohol, and drugs at the same time were more than 11× more likely to die by suicide.

There were also significant gender differences. Women with multiple addictions – tobacco, alcohol, and drugs – were more than 16 times as likely to die by suicide as women without addictions. In men, having the same combination of addictions increased the risk of dying by suicide by about 8 times.

Addiction appears to interact with biology and gender factors, being more damaging to women but potentially more common in men.

According to the Men's Health Forum in the UK: [40]

"Men are nearly three times more likely than women to become alcohol dependent (8.7% of men are alcohol dependent compared to 3.3% of women)."

And when it comes to drugs: *"Men are three times as likely to report frequent drug use than women (4.2% and 1.4% respectively) and more than two thirds of drug-related deaths occur in men."*

A study published in *Journal of Behavioral Addictions* in 2019 found that men are 3.5× more likely to agree with the statement *"I am addicted to pornography"* than women are (11% of men vs 3% of women). [41]

Maybe it's no coincidence that men are 3× more likely to be addicted to alcohol, 3× more likely to use recreational drugs, 3.5× more likely identify as addicted to porn, *and* 3× more likely to die from suicide than women?

When I first learned this, I wondered what it is about addictions that makes them so dangerous when it comes to their associated risk with suicide. Of course, there is the obvious aftermath that can result from any addiction: financial, social, and relationship destruction. But then there is a biological element: people suffering from addictions are often more impulsive. And impulsivity is strongly associated with suicide. [42] [43]

So addiction, impulsivity, and suicide all seem to share a relationship. But is this correlation or causation? One of the reasons I believe this relationship exists is because of the effect that addictive substances have on our brains.

We know that dopamine is triggered by novelty. But it also makes us want to seek out more novelty. This means there needs to be a safety switch to keep things balanced. Without this, a novelty–dopamine feedback loop could spiral out of control. Mammals would become impulsive, roaming miles from the safety of their home in search of new things. Luckily, we have a natural safety switch inside our brains that prevents this from happening.

When dopamine is released in your brain – let's say you are doing something holistic like a workout or getting a morning walk – it hits many different kinds of receptors. Two of these receptors are known as D1 and D2 receptors. Their roles are extremely complicated, but in general: [44]

- D1 receptors are associated with motivation
- D2 receptors are associated with restraint

The balance between D1 and D2 receptors is extremely important. If the D1 receptors were to overpower the D2 receptors, it could be like the accelerator pedal getting stuck in your car.

In animal studies, consistently giving cocaine to mice reduces the D2 receptors associated with restraint, making them more impulsive. This broken balance continues after the initial dopamine "spike" has passed. The more used to cocaine the mice are, the longer this impulsive period lasts. [45]

Like the mice, in human studies, it's been found that people who are addicted to drugs also have reduced D2 receptors. This is all extremely oversimplified, but it suggests that addictive substances have a wider effect on our overall decision-making and impulsivity. [46] This could explain why some drugs seem to act as "gateway drugs", changing our decision-making and normalising more extreme, more damaging drugs.

I've found that some people don't like this theory. They don't like to think a substance could change their brain and, ultimately, change the decisions they make. But many people experience this in their everyday lives. Including people with – or caring for those with – Parkinson's disease.

Parkinson's is a condition that primarily affects movement. You know now that dopamine in the brain is associated with movement. Parkinson's is due to when these dopamine-producing cells die off, resulting in symptoms like tremors and rigidity.

Medication used to manage Parkinson's disease imitates dopamine ("*dopamine agonists*"), compensating for the low dopamine activity in the brain. By doing this, the medication can provide significant symptom relief and help to maintain quality of life. But as the medication is essentially manipulating dopamine production, it can also cause strong impulsive behaviour.

To quote The Parkinson's Foundation:

"*Impulse control behaviors (ICBs) affect between 14% and 40% of people with Parkinson's disease (PD). Examples of ICB's include compulsive gambling or shopping, hoarding and hyper sexuality. [...] Only 2% of people have ICBs in the general population. Why the dramatic disparity? It has to do with the gold standard medication for PD: Dopamine replacement therapy, such as L-dopa, as well as [medications which imitate dopamine], are all strongly linked to experiencing ICBs.*" [47]

To quote another of their articles:

"*Scientists have known for over a decade that dopamine-related drugs for Parkinson's could be linked to impulse control disorders (ICDs). However, it was not until 2004 that people living with Parkinson's began to learn that ICDs could be a rare side effect of [medications which imitate dopamine]. Today, we know that one in six people taking [this kind of medication] will experience ICDs.*"

"*For some people, ICDs may be mild, or just a minor nuisance (for example, increased focus on eating sweets). For others, the impact may be more severe. People who experience compulsive gambling and compulsive shopping may lose large sums of money, even to the point of bankruptcy. Those* who binge eat may experience significant weight gain, causing discomfort and embarrassment and possibly increasing vascular disease risk factors. Some of those who experience compulsive sexual behaviors may begin engaging in unprotected sex or sex outside of an established relationship, placing themselves and others at risk physically and emotionally. ICDs typically impact not only the person living with Parkinson's disease, but loved ones as well."* [48]

I'm not sharing this information to discourage anyone with Parkinson's from using medication that can help them to manage their symptoms and improve their quality of life. The only reason I am sharing these articles from The Parkinson's Foundation is because I believe that there is a lesson we can learn from the experiences of people with Parkinson's disease and caring for those with Parkinson's disease. **Things that impact our dopamine system impact our impulsivity and decision-making.**

This could also be true of addictive behaviours, not just substances. According to one article:

"Studies show that addictive behaviors can produce brain changes corresponding to drug use, sometimes with a reduction in the electrical activity of the prefrontal region, an area responsible for assessing potential risks and inhibiting impulsivity." [49]

This matters because — beyond the concerning link with suicide — anything that affects our dopamine system can make us more impulsive. This can undermine the decision-making and discipline needed to make positive life changes.

While most people would probably not identify with having an addiction, I believe that most of us can identify with having 'distractions' in our lives. Whether it's alcohol, social media, porn, or video games, many of us have certain things that take us away from enjoying more important and healthier experiences.

Which brings me on to the most important part of this section: what in the world are we meant to do about it?

Restoring motivation and discipline

The online meeting began. I was in my home office and Christopher was in a hotel room in Croatia, filming the second season of the historical drama he had been cast in when we first worked together 2 years before. We had stayed in touch throughout his journey, and we tended to work together each time he was preparing for a new major role.

He gave me a brief tour of the hotel room. Out of the window, his hotel overlooked white yachts mooring next to golden cliffs in the blue Adriatic Sea. He was still living the adventure he described in the Future Call from our first coaching call together.

"What's on your mind?" I asked as he sat back down again.

Christopher pulled a face as if someone had just stepped on his toe. He ran his hand through his thick brown hair and looked out of the balcony and at the horizon. Then he buried his face with both hands and slammed his elbows down onto the table in his hotel room. He froze for a moment, head in his hands. His shoulders rose and fell with a loud sigh.

"I knew I had four days between shoots. *Four days.* That was time dedicated to writing the script I have been thinking about for months. Once these four days finish, I'm back to shooting for weeks with almost no time to work on the script. This was my chance to write the script. It's the morning of *day three*, and I haven't even started. *Haven't... Even... Started...*"

His right hand now tugged at the collar of his white cheesecloth shirt in frustration, then fell lifelessly to the table, with a thud. He didn't wince or blink, but let out another disappointed sigh.

"What are the main things holding you back from working on your script?" I asked, helping him to identify the main obstacles.

"Honestly, man? It's mainly Netflix... I keep telling myself that watching good dramas on Netflix is work, but it really isn't. Creating *my own script* is work, not watching other peoples'. The trouble is this—"

Christopher spun around and stretched an arm to an enormous TV screen on the hotel wall behind him. The blue glow of the cloudless Croatian sky reflected in its black mirror. It was quite a contrast.

"And what else?" I continued.

"Yeah, also my phone. Well, not my phone, but WhatsApp. I keep checking it to see whether the lads from set are heading out to do anything, so I don't miss out. The thing is, they're not going out. I'm just wasting my time looking at chats and making small talk. Then, this morning I was just scrolling through Instagram Reels. Instagram Reels! My brain is screaming, '*What's wrong with you, man? You have this one shot to write your own script while you are on a BBC set, and you're bingeing on Netflix, WhatsApp, and Instagram like you do when you're back at home with nothing to do!*' I almost wouldn't mind if I'd been off exploring the location. But I haven't even done that."

I waited until I was sure that Christopher had identified all his obstacles. Then I asked my next question:

"If you had hired a scriptwriter for four days to write a script for you, and he was getting distracted by Netflix, WhatsApp, and Instagram, what would you do to help him?"

"Easy," he said, with an open hand – as if it was the stupidest question in the whole world. "I would say, '*C'mon, man, we're here to write, not to doomscroll.*' And I would unplug the TV from the wall... And I would take the batteries out of the remote control. Just stop those distractions from..."

His words faded and we sat looking at one another, through our cameras. A thousand miles apart, but there together. His eyebrows raised. He stood up in silence and disappeared into the background of the room. I heard the clicking of switches and the unplugging of plugs.

When he came back into view, Christopher opened a hand and dropped 2 silver batteries onto the table. "Done. What next?"

"What if your scriptwriter told you he was being distracted by his WhatsApp? And his friends?"

Christopher reached for his phone and began typing into it. "It's simple," he said. "Tell your friends..." (It looked like he was typing as he said the words to me)

"*'Hi guys, taking the day to work on my script. Tell you about it later. I won't be on WhatsApp but if you are going out tonight, give me a knock on my hotel door after eight p.m. But until then, I need to focus. Cheers, Christopher.'*" Still imagining himself speaking to his scriptwriter, he said, "Now put your phone into airplane mode. Or, better yet, just turn it off."

He held the lock and volume buttons on his phone, turning it off with a swipe. Then he opened a drawer in the table and dropped the phone in there like it was rubbish going into a bin. He pushed the drawer shut.

I followed up with: "What next?". I could feel the momentum building.

"OK," he instructed himself. "You have to open Google Sheets, hit 'File' and then 'Make available offline'. Now you don't have to be online to work on your script. The downside is you probably can't use voice-to-text, but the plus side is, no distractions."

"And what else?" I asked.

Christopher stared again out of the balcony. I waited in silence while he slowly sighed several times. I didn't want to interrupt, because coming up with his own solutions is often the most valuable way he can spend his time. It's the most powerful part of coaching – and supporting men in general.

"No, that's it," he eventually shared. "Netflix is gone… The TV is unplugged… The phone and the laptop can't interrupt me… Can I tell you something really strange?"

"Of course you can."

"It feels like, now those distractions are gone… Now there is nothing to do but to work on my script. It kind of feels as if all that focus that was going into Netflix is now being directed into my script. Not being rude, but I kind of feel like I need to get off this call and go work on my script…"

"Perfect. What accountability would you like from me?"

"Tomorrow…" Christopher said. "I'll call you tomorrow at eight a.m. UK time. I need you to ask me: 'How many words did you type yesterday?' And do the same the next day too. That plus no distractions will help me to make the most of these two days."

"Deal. Go and write your script, man."

Christopher wrote 6,500 words that day, and 7,000 words the following day. In the 12 months prior, he had thought about his script every day, but written 0 words. Our call was short but effective: we just had to identify and remove the cues that led to his distractions.

Before this section ends, I want to share 2 concepts with you that some of my clients have found helpful in understanding dopamine. These aren't scientific models, more like oversimplified concepts we can use in our life.

Concept #1: 'Shut the Door' to Distractions

This is what enabled Christopher to work on his script. Dopamine is triggered by cues in our environment. Signs that we have an opportunity to do something that was previously rewarding. This means that sights, smells, and situations that previously led to a dopamine spike can trigger cravings and automatic behaviours. By deactivating his TV, remote, phone, and laptop, Christopher removed these cues from his environment. This is a great way to overcome distractions without replying upon willpower.

Here are some ways that men I have worked with have Shut the Door to previous distractions or addictions:

- Sugar cravings: have no sugar in the house, only stock healthy food.
- Recreational drugs: don't hang around with people who are using drugs, don't go to places where drugs are available, delete dealer's number from phone.
- Gambling: register for self exclusion – in the UK this has been done with multiple different schemes, depending on the type of gambling you want to be excluded from. They are all listed on the Betting & Gaming Council's "Self Exclusion" page. [50]

For clarity, I am not suggesting that we all need to stop doing anything that vaguely resembles enjoyment. But shutting the door is an important strategy to be able to remove distractions or harmful behaviours when needed.

For example, I enjoy watching YouTube videos, and wouldn't want to stop that for the rest of my life. But I also know that this book would never have been finished if I had not decided to stop watching YouTube until this book was completed. So that I wasn't relying on willpower, I used the Freedom app to block YouTube (both the app and URL) on all my devices. This was a key part of me "finding the time" to write this book and closing the door to anything that might get in the way of that.

Concept #2: The Hard Reset

A Hard Reset means cutting out a distraction or addiction for at least 90 days. Certain addictions can cause physical dependencies that would cause harm if you went cold turkey, so expert help may be needed in those situations. That's why one of the questions in my D-10 Questionnaire (you'll see later) is *"Would it be difficult / dangerous to give up without the right help?"* There are other tools that can be used to assess how safe it is to stop. For example, the UK site DrinkAware.co.uk has tools to help you to identify the risk of alcohol dependence, plan ways to cut down, and plan ways to stop.

Assuming it is safe for men to "cut out" a distraction or addiction, their experience always seems to follow a very similar pattern.

Time into the Hard Reset	Typical comments from Clients
Day 1	*"It's going to be difficult."*
Day 21	*"I'm feeling the benefit."*
Day 90	*"It's easy. I don't know why I worried."*
Day 180	*"I don't think I'll ever go back."*

In coaching, men regularly tell me that cutting out something they previously found distracting has been beneficial for their motivation, discipline, and decision-making. There isn't much research into this, but small experiments have found that cutting out things – from a favourite food to pornography – led to people being able to delay other forms of gratification for greater goals. That's ultimately what we are trying to do and the reason why it might be useful to cut out certain distractions. [51]

A hard reset doesn't have to be forever. But after 90 days without something, we are in a strong position to decide whether we want to re-introduce it to our lives, without cravings clouding our judgement.

Having Adventures: Strategies

Having Adventures is about feeling motivated and disciplined. In this part of the book, we have explored how many substances and activities impact the brain's dopamine systems, causing impulsivity and potential addiction which are associated with higher risk of suicide. We also explored the protective role of cutting out distractions. We can all support the men we care about by simply by supporting them to take breaks from work, routine, and distractions.

❏ Take time to 'recharge'

Some men are particularly bad at taking time away from their day-to-day routine. This isn't limited to their official "holiday", but that can be part of it. A rule that has served some of my clients well is the "Rolling Holiday" rule. This is where you don't return to work without booking another break of the equivalent length.

Let's say I had just returned from a 7-day holiday that used 5 days of annual leave: I would have to pencil in another 5 days off before returning to work. The details don't have to be arranged, but this placeholder in the diary gives me something to work towards and prevents me from getting "too busy" to take time off in the future.

You don't have to be on holiday or spend any money to recharge your batteries. In my coaching programme, I ask men "What recharges your battery?" It has to be things that (1) make them feel energised again and (2) they don't regret afterwards. This has led to all kinds of answers, including:

"walking my dog in the woods", "painting miniature soldiers", "tinkering with my car", or "riding my motorbike". Once we have identified what charges his batteries, the next step is to set the time aside to actually do it. That can be where accountability comes in. Just ask the question: "What accountability would you like from me?" Maybe no accountability is needed. Maybe it will make all the difference to him.

❏ Explore new places and skills

Is there a place or a skill that he, you, or both of you have been wanting to explore? Now is the time to do it. Novelty and variety release dopamine in our brains, boosting motivation and creating those positive lasting memories. In an ideal world, we would all be aware of the need for variety and take the initiative to ensure we get it. But not everyone is experienced at planning adventures. If you are in a position to do so, take the lead and invite him along, or find someone else who is in a position to do so.

❏ Identify distractions

In my coaching practice, I have developed a tool called the D-10 Questionnaire. It's a useful tool for identifying when a potential distraction might be causing issues in life, and I generally find that men are quite keen to use it. It is not a clinical or diagnostic tool, just some thoughtful questions that can help with self-awareness and personal reflection.

The way it works is you pick something that you feel might be distracting you in life (alcohol, social media, or internet porn, etc.) and you replace the 'x' in each sentence with the thing you want to test:

The D-10 Questionnaire

Q1 ⇒ Do you look forward to x while you are doing other things?

Q2 ⇒ Do you find yourself doing x for longer than intended?

Q3 ⇒ Do you use x to "unwind" or escape from problems?

Q4 ⇒ Does x distract you from doing healthier or more important things?

Q5 ⇒ Have you tried to cut down on x before but found it difficult?

Q6 ⇒ Do you need more x now than you used to?

Q7 ⇒ Does the idea of giving up x make you feel uncomfortable or anxious?

Q8 ⇒ Do you ever regret how much time or money you spend on x?

Q9 ⇒ Have you lied to others about how much you use x?

Q10 ⇒ Would it be difficult or dangerous to give up x without the right help?

There is no "pass" or "fail" score, but it can be valuable to pay attention to any "yes" answers because they could represent ways that this distraction is having a negative impact. The questions are based around dopamine dysregulation. Question 10 is a safeguarding question, designed to help men to realise when expert help might be needed.

❑ Cut out / get help with distractions

If someone you care about is performing a Hard Reset, do you have to do it with them? My opinion is that you don't, but there are some things you can do to make it easier for them.

I have helped many men give up smoking cigarettes. It didn't matter that I wasn't also giving them up (because I have never smoked). What they wanted from me was regular check-ins and accountability. But it would probably have been harder for them if I joined the accountability call each morning with a cigarette in my mouth.

The snag often crops up when you live together. It's hard to be the only one in your house who gives something up – you can't just "shut the door" and so you have to rely on a lot of willpower. Particularly when it comes to giving up alcohol and following low-carbohydrate diets, it is often a family member who convinces men to break their Hard Reset with "*just one beer*" or "*just one Coke*". This might seem harmless, but it defeats the purpose of what that man is trying to achieve. Where you can, support Hard Resets and celebrate their importance.

Where he needs support beyond accountability (for example, from specialists like addiction or medical experts) you can help by reframing it as 'teaming up' with experts to grow his understanding, skills, and confidence. You can also assist with practical steps, such as researching services, or — if it feels right — attending the initial appointments. Of course, your relationship and instincts will be your best guide.

❏ Use smartphone in black and white mode

These are many reasons to believe that smartphones dysregulate our dopamine systems. Thankfully, there are many quick changes that you can make so your smartphone is less distracting and addictive. The single most important change you can make is using it in black and white.

By removing the sharp, contrasting colour, you reduce the way it stimulates dopamine in your brain. This is an excellent way to prevent your phone from stealing your attention and motivation. Not only will this improve your life, but by modelling this behaviour, you can also make a difference to the men you care about too.

A word of warning though: when you first try it, you may hate it! That's because your phone has been stimulating your dopamine system for years. But if you can stick with it for a few days, you will feel the benefit!

Phone menus are always changing, so head to the Resources page on my website and I will keep an updated video on how to turn on this black and white mode, plus any other changes you can make to ensure your phone is still perfectly usable in this mode.

Share this with the men in your life, but first make sure you are using it yourself!

Ultimately, our aim is to empower the men we care about to take breaks from routine, tackle distractions, and create positive memories along the way. This becomes much easier when we understand how dopamine drives motivation, focus, and distraction. These five strategies have helped many of my clients strengthen their discipline, boost their motivation, and slow down the pace of life.

ENDNOTES

1. I later learned that "swell" like this can roll in from far-off storms, meaning high waves can last long after the local wind has died. One source that explains this is R1541: The Royal National Lifeboat Institution (2020). "The science of waves." RNLI.org.
2. R1354: M Richardson (2019). "How much energy does the brain use?" BrainFacts.org.
3. R1433: P Atchley, S Lane (2014). "Chapter Four - Cognition in the attention economy." Psychology of Learning and Motivation.
4. R1502: Cedars Sinai (2018). "Study sheds light on how 'dopamine neurons' contribute to memory formation in humans." cedars-sinai.org.
5. R1308: A Duszkiewicz et al. (2019). "Novelty and dopaminergic modulation of memory persistence: A tale of two systems." Trends in Neuroscience.
6. I've simplified a lot here. I am talking here about how dopamine travels through the mesolimbic, mesocortical and nigrostriatal pathways, stimulating the nucleus accumbens (NAc), striatum, hippocampus, and amygdala in the brain.
7. I know 462 drives to work might sound like a lot, but it's only 2 years of working days, minus 22 days of holiday and 8 public UK holidays a year.
8. R1356: T Hills (2006). "Animal foraging and the evolution of goal-directed cognition." Cognitive Science.
9. R1325: V Costa et al. (2014). "Dopamine modulates novelty seeking behavior during decision making." Behavioral Neuroscience.
10. The explanation of how cocaine impacts you is a combination of my understanding of addictive substances, combined with a detailed article: R1345: G Koob & N Volkow (2010). "Neurocircuitry of addiction." Neuropsychopharmacology.
11. R1335: N Volkow et al. (2010). "Addiction: Beyond dopamine reward circuitry." The Proceedings of the National Academy of Sciences.
12. R1314: R Wise (2009). "Roles for nigrostriatal—not just mesocorticolimbic—dopamine in reward and addiction." Trends in Neurosciences.
13. R1343: K Park et al. (2013). "Chronic cocaine dampens dopamine signaling during cocaine intoxication and unbalances D1 over D2 receptor signaling." Journal of Neuroscience.
14. R1523: National Institute on Drug Abuse, NIDA (2025). "Drugs, brains, and behavior: The science of addiction." nida.nih.gov.
15. Again, this chapter contains lots of references to information that is very well summarised in R1345: G Koob & N Volkow (2010). "Neurocircuitry of addiction." Neuropsychopharmacology.
16. R1549: H Boecker et al (2008). "The Runner's High: Opioidergic Mechanisms in the Human Brain." Cerebral Cortex.
17. R1550: D Raichlen et al (2012). "Wired to run: exercise-induced endocannabinoid signaling in humans and cursorial mammals with implications for the 'runner's high'." Journal of Experimental Biology.
18. R1427: The National Archives (Accessed 2025). "Psychoactive Substances Act 2016." legislation.gov.uk.

19 R1347: B Lennerz et al. (2013). "Effects of dietary glycemic index on brain regions related to reward and craving in men." The American Journal of Clinical Nutrition.
20 R1348: B Lennerz et al. (2018). "Food addiction, high-glycemic-index carbohydrates, and obesity." Clinical Chemistry.
21 R1349: L Pruimboom et al. (2015). "The opioid effects of gluten exorphins: asymptomatic celiac disease." Journal of Health Population and Nutrition.
22 R1350: M R U Haq (2020). "Structure and production of casomorphins." Opioid Food Peptides.
23 R1552: J Hilliard et al (Accessed 2025). "Loperamide Addiction and Abuse." Addiction Center.
24 Both exorphins and Loperamide act upon μ-opioid receptors in the gut (pronounced "mu-opioid").
25 R850: M A Proll et al. (1982). "Use of liquid chromatography with electrochemistry to measure effects of varying intensities of white light on DOPA accumulation in rat retinas." Life Sciences.
26 R1351: Apple.com (Accessed 2025). "iPhone 16 - Tech Specs." support.apple.com.
27 Here's how I calculated the '1,400 lux' estimate: iPhone brightness is given in nits (how much brightness the screen emits), but we want to know lux (how much brightness actually reaches the eye). The standard maximum brightness is 1,000 nits. I assumed indoor use at 50% brightness, held 45 cm from the face, and various AI tools estimated around 1,396 lux. However, any calculation converting nits to lux is hypothetical, and different methods can produce very different results. It's also worth noting that the rats in the animal study had been kept in the dark beforehand, which may have made them more sensitive to light. Despite these caveats, I've included this paragraph to highlight the potential for phone screens to influence our dopamine system — and the surprising lack of research into this.
28 R414: L-C Wickord et al. (2023). "Suffering from problematic smartphone use? Why not use grayscale setting as an intervention! – An experimental study." Computers in Human Behavior Reports.
29 Also called "Intermittent Reinforcement" in behavioural psychology and "Intermittent Reward Scheduling" in gaming and app design.
30 R1352: SEMRUSH (Accessed 2025). "Most visited websites in the United Kingdom, updated March 2025." Semrush.com.
31 R1504: Jeff Orlowski, Davis Coombe and Vickie Curtis (2020). The Social Dilemma. Netflix Original.
32 R847: B Park et al. (2016). "Is internet pornography causing sexual dysfunctions? A review with clinical reports." Behavioral Science.
33 R1202: H Garavan et al. (2000). "Cue-induced cocaine craving: neuroanatomical specificity for drug users and drug stimuli." The American Journal of Psychiatry.
34 R847: B Park et al. (2016).
35 R847: B Park et al. (2016).
36 R1200: S Perry (2016). "Does viewing pornography reduce marital quality over time? Evidence from longitudinal data." Archives of Sexual Behavior.

37 R1201: S Perry (2017). "Pornography use and marital separation: Evidence from two-wave panel data." Archives of Sexual Behavior.
38 R847: B Park et al. (2016). "Is internet pornography causing sexual dysfunctions? A review with clinical reports." Behavioral Science.
39 R1428: F Lynch et al. (2020). "Substance use disorders and risk of suicide in a general US population: a case control study." Addiction Science & Clinical Practice.
40 R406: Men's Health Forum (2017). "Key data: Mental health." menshealthforum.org.uk.
41 R1191: J Grubbs et al. (2019). "Self-reported addiction to pornography in a nationally representative sample: The roles of use habits, religiousness, and moral incongruence." Journal of Behavioral Addictions.
42 R1505: American Society of Addiction Medicine (2021). "On impulsivity: The neuroscience of behavior associated with addiction." ASAM.org.
43 R1429: R Liu et al. (2017). "A behavioral and cognitive neuroscience perspective on impulsivity, suicide, and non-suicidal self-injury: Meta-analysis and recommendations for future research." Neuroscience & Biobehavioral Reviews.
44 R1333: I Kawahata et al. (2024). "Dopamine D1–D5 receptors in brain nuclei: implications for health and disease." Receptors.
45 R1343: K Park et al. (2013). "Chronic cocaine dampens dopamine signaling during cocaine intoxication and unbalances D1 over D2 receptor signaling." Journal of Neuroscience.
46 R1345: G Koob & N Volkow (2010). "Neurocircuitry of addiction." Neuropsychopharmacology.
47 R1430: The Parkinson's Foundation (Accessed 2025). "New study examines impulse control, REM sleep and dopamine." parkinson.org.
48 R1431: The Parkinson's Foundation (Accessed 2025). "Impulse control." parkinson.org.
49 R1447: D Malagone de Albuquerque et al. (2023). "Dopaminergic pathways and their addictions: gambling on dopamine." International Seven Journal of Multidisciplinary (translated into English for the Semantic Scholar corpus).
50 R1432: Betting & Gaming Council (Accessed 2025). "Self exclusion schemes." bettingandgamingcouncil.com/sense-self-exclusion-scheme.
51 R424: S Negash et al. (2015). "Trading later rewards for current pleasure: Pornography consumption and delay discounting." The Journal of Sex Research.

PART 6

ABLE TO SERVE

> *"Life is never made unbearable by circumstances, but only by lack of meaning and purpose."*
>
> – Victor Frankl

Able to Serve	
Signs of stress	• Feeling *useless* • Feeling *unfulfilled* • Wondering *what is the point of life?* • Loss of child contact • Death feels meaningful or *heroic*

Jaden's story

Jaden is good-looking and well-built. Despite being out of the US Army for 3 years, he sports a standard issue military style buzz haircut and his impressive biceps are framed by a tight black T-shirt with the word 'ARMY' on it. This is his Future Call:

Jaden's Future Call

Ryan: Ring-ring! Ring-right. Hi, Jaden, I wasn't expecting your call. How are you doing?

Jaden: Holy crap, Ryan. My life is so good right now, I just called to tell you about it… Basically, I kept doing what was working for me, but I also made some specific changes to my life, based around the Framework we discussed. When it came to Achieving Recognition, brother, I always had what I needed. When I was in the army I made it my business to progress through the ranks as quickly as I could. I could always see a way to make it to the next level. And when I went for a job on civvy street, I did the same thing. Set small goals, put in the effort. Get that sense of progress. And when it came to Looking After Body & Mind, I've always been good at that. I still start my days with a morning run, then I get in my weights session, working all major muscle groups. I follow a drill they taught us when I was stateside. It really works for me, and I've carried on doing that this last year. So there's been no change there really.

Ryan: That's great, Jaden, well done for recognising the areas where you were already doing so well. How about Protecting the Cave? What's your financial situation like now?

Jaden: Yeah, that's one where I needed to make some changes. So last year, I was earning good money but I used to always spend more than I earned. I was blasting away all my money on things I didn't need. And I really got that under control.

Ryan: What did you decide to do about it?

Jaden: When we met last year, I realised that because of my time in the army, I had never really learned to manage money. My accommodation and food was always catered for. So my wages were just for spending. I carried on that mindset when I came over here, and that caused me a lot of problems."

Ryan: How about Having Adventures? Where were you twelve months ago and what's that like now?

Jaden: Oh yeah, that's much better now. That technique we spoke about – giving my partner permission to book holidays – really worked. My holiday was used up before I could say 'Thank you!'

[By this point, Jaden was in a positive mood and he was firing out solutions. He was warmed up and ready for the final 5 questions. What came out of it was a big surprise...]

Ryan: Cast your mind back to when we had that very first Zoom call together, at the time, what was the main thing that was holding you back?

Jaden: Oh it was... It was not being able to see my daughter Aimee. You see, I didn't tell you but the reason why my partner and I moved to London was because my ex-wife moved my daughter over here, to be with her family. And I can't describe the pain to you, brother. Not being able to see your little girl, it's like a knife in your heart. The idea that she's growing up without me. That she doesn't know me. That I don't know her. Brother, it's more than I could take. And that is why I was spending my money on stupid shit. I just had to do something to numb the pain and deal with the thoughts in my head. The pain of not seeing Aimee.

Ryan: What did you do to overcome the pain and become who you wanted to be?

Jaden: Well, I would love to tell you that things changed, and she's allowed to see me now. But that's just not the way that things work. So here's what I did first... I decided to focus on what I can control. I couldn't control whether Aimee's mum lets me see her. But I could control what I did with my time... and my money. And so, each week when I got paid, I would set the evening aside. And I would write a letter to my little girl. Yeah, brother, I would write her a real, handwritten letter. And I would tell her how much I loved her, how I thought of her all week, and how I couldn't wait to see the young woman that she is becoming. Then I copied the letter. I posted one copy to her mum's address, and I kept the other in my apartment. And then... the money I used to waste on gadgets and stupid things to fill the hole in my heart, I invested it for her. Yeah... At first I had no idea what to get, so I bought a gold coin, sort of like an investment. And I kept it for her. Each week when I got paid, I'd write her a little letter, copy the letter, and buy her another gold coin. I hope that her mum is passing the letters on to her. But if not, I know one day she'll come find me. And when she does, I'll be able to share with her all the letters, all the gold coins, and all the love from all my years without her. And she'll know that everything I did, I did for her. She'll know that I loved her all along. And if that's all I get... Man, I will endure anything for that. I will walk across broken glass in bare feet just for the opportunity to give Aimee those letters and that money. And she'll know that I loved her all along!

[Tears streamed down Jaden's face. I had to clear my throat before I could continue.]

Ryan: You are quite a man, Jaden. And you're an amazing father. You've had an amazing year, but I want to know: what has been the single best thing you've done all year?

Jaden: I made myself useful. I stopped talking about the pain and focussed on what would make the pain worth enduring. I dealt with it by building a future for Aimee. I put my love and my wisdom into those letters, in a way that my father never did for me. I became the father figure I never had.

Ryan: If I had a time machine, and you could send a message back in time to be delivered to Jaden at the end of his first coaching session one year ago, what would you say to him? What did he need to hear at the time?

Jaden: I would say... *"Jaden, man. Aimee needs her dad. She needs you, man. You might not be able to see her and to watch her grow. But you can still be ready for her when the time comes. And when she comes for you, she'll see that you would walk through fire and across broken glass just to give her the letters and that investment you made for her. And she'll know that you were thinking of her all along. That you loved her all along."*

Ryan: It's been an absolute honour seeing what you've achieved over the past year Jaden, but I want to know... Cast your mind back to that first coaching session we had a year ago. I want to know: what was the very first thing you did after that session that got this amazing year off to a great start?

Jaden: I bought that first little coin for Aimee... For my daughter's future... Then I sat down with a pen, turned off all the distractions in my life, and I wrote my first letter to my little girl. And I told her about all the plans that her dad has for her future. And I told her I will wait forever for the day we meet again.

Ryan: Wow... Jaden. You've had an amazing year and it's been my honour to see you take control of the things which you could. I know there were times where you made use of the expertise of others – your partner, money mentors, and all the people who have helped you along the way – but ultimately *YOU* made this happen. You realised what would make the pain worth bearing and you committed to it. I know your partner's proud of you, I'm proud of you, and you should be proud of yourself. Because one day soon, your daughter will be proud of you too.

Jaden: Thank you, brother. For her... I can never stop.

Ryan: I have to go now, but it was great catching up.

Jaden: Thank you, man. Thank you.

Ryan: Goodbye, Jaden.
BEEP

At the point of writing this book, Jaden has not yet been reunited with Aimee. But he continues to write to her, and he continues to save for her. The idea of Aimee knocking on his door one day gives Jaden a sense of purpose.

The final A in ALPHA stands for **Able to Serve**. It's about the things men need to do for their sense of purpose.

Able to Serve: The science

It's not a lack of talking or talking therapy

Read most articles about male mental health in the UK media, and there are 2 figures that keep coming up:

- Around 75% of UK deaths from suicide are men
- Only 36% of UK referrals to talking therapy are for men

These 2 facts being positioned so closely together makes it seem as if they are related. I know that many people hear this and assume that *"75% of deaths from suicide are men **because** not enough men are being referred to talking therapy."*

This, combined with the experience that men are less likely to talk about feelings than women, can lead people to think, *"If men were willing to attend talking therapy and talk about they feel, the rate of suicide in men would be lower."*

But is it as simple as that?

One of the most basic fallacies (things that sound logical but aren't) is to see things together and assume that one must be causing the other. But these 2 facts, presented together, are not only oversimplified, they may also be misleading.

One of the many things that this equation completely neglects to mention is that **women are more likely to think about suicide, and more likely to attempt suicide,** than men.[1][2][3][4]

The reason why men are more likely to die from suicide is not because they are more likely to attempt suicide, it's because they use more lethal methods to end their lives.[5]

But there are other reasons why someone might seek talking therapy, besides thoughts about suicide. According to a 2017 report by the Mental Health Foundation, women are 3× more likely to experience common mental health problems than men, 3× more likely to experience eating disorders than men, and 3× more likely to experience post-traumatic stress disorder (PTSD) than men. When you take this into account, 36% of referrals to talking therapy being men doesn't seem that low... [6]

So rather than comparing women with men, let's instead compare men of today with men of the recent past. And in many ways, men are more open today.

In their 2022 Public Perceptions Survey, the British Association for Counselling and Psychotherapy (BACP) found that, compared with 5 years before (2017): [7]

- 79% of men agree it's more socially acceptable to discuss mental health
- 69% of men say they're more aware of mental health issues
- 68% of men say there's less of a stigma around mental health

These are all good things to see.

The BACP also found that between 2010 and 2022, the rate of men who had been for talking therapy had increased by 50% (from 18% in 2010 to 27% in 2022). That's a massive difference. In fact, it appears from the BACP's survey that things are getting better for men.

But, in the same time that UK men have become 50% more likely to attend talking therapy, they have also become 14% more likely to die from suicide, according to the Office for National Statistics. [8]

And when you compare different age groups of men, Samaritans found that the peak of professional support use is in middle age, with older and younger men more reluctant to reach out for help. And which age group of men dies at the highest rate of suicide? Middle-aged men. The ones who are the most open to getting formal support. [9]

So it appears that:

- When you compare men to women, the sex that uses talking therapy the most (women) attempts suicide the most.

- When you compare men of 2010 with men of 2022, the men who use talking therapy the most (men in 2022) have the higher rates of suicide.
- When you compare different age groups of men, the age group of men that uses formal support the most (middle-aged men) has the highest rate of suicide.

Now, before anyone says *"correlation isn't causation"* — I know that. But here's the issue: the same people who say to me *"correlation isn't causation"* when I share these statistics are often the ones who just said: *"75% of suicides are men, and yet men make up only 36% of referrals to talking therapy."* In doing so, they suggest that these 2 are linked. There's a double standard here.

Above all, I am not trying to discourage anyone from talking therapy — why would I? My aim is simply to show that the situation is more complex than a simple lack of talking therapy. We need to think critically, because oversimplified explanations will fail to help the men who are most at risk.

In the UK's 2017 National Confidential Inquiry into Suicide and Safety in Mental Health (the last time I reference it, I promise), it was found that:

"Almost all (91%) middle-aged men [who died from suicide] had been in contact with at least one frontline service or agency, most often primary care services (82%). Half had been in contact with mental health services, 30% with the justice system.

"It is therefore too simplistic to say men do not seek help. We should focus on how services can improve the recognition of risk and respond to men's needs, and how services might work better together." [10]

And in the words of the Hope project (the mental health service in Bristol that addresses male suicide by helping men to address financial issues):

"Mental health, emotional wellbeing and suicide are all topics more freely discussed today than ever before. Yet one in five of us will have suicidal thoughts and every 90 minutes someone will end their life." [11]

In my experience, normally when men reach out for formal support with their mental health, they are referred to talking therapy and prescribed antidepressants – just like Brad was. So the next question we need to ask is: what impact do these things have on thoughts about suicide in men?

Why the current approach might not be enough to tackle male suicide

In a 2012 report, Samaritans warned that:

"Generic 'talking' therapy may not be effective for 'at risk' men, because [...] the specific psychological factors generating their suicidality are not being addressed." [12]

This might be surprising for some people to read, but you may be even more surprised to learn there isn't a great deal of research into how effective talking therapy is for those having thoughts about suicide. An article published in *Depression and Anxiety* in 2021 stated that:

"A recent meta-analysis examining the effects of psychotherapy for depressed adults found that only 3 out of 1,344 studies reported outcomes related to suicidal cognitions or behaviors. In these studies, the effect of treatments on suicidal ideation and suicide risk was small and nonsignificant." [13]

The article explained that talking therapy can help to tackle thoughts about suicide, when that therapy is focussed on thoughts about suicide. But current guidelines mean that people who are having thoughts about suicide are given talking therapy designed to help with depression.

The article continues:

"Currently, the two most commonly practiced psychological treatments for depression are cognitive behavior therapy (CBT) and interpersonal psychotherapy (IPT). [...] For now, there is insufficient trial evidence to suggest that CBT for depression also leads to reduced suicidal cognitions and behaviors. Even less evidence is available on the efficacy of IPT in reducing [thoughts about suicide]."

The recent meta-analysis which this article was talking about was carried out by Prof (Dr) Pim Cuijpers and his team (mainly) from the Department of Clinical Psychology, Vrije Universiteit in Amsterdam. Prof Cuijpers' study concluded with the words:

"At this point, there is insufficient evidence for the assumption that suicidality in depressed patients can be reduced with psychotherapy for depression. Although psychotherapy of depression may have small positive effects on suicidality, available data suggest that psychotherapy for depression cannot be considered to be a sufficient treatment." [14]

In 2018, an article published in *Psychiatric Times* warned that many clinicians wrongly believe that treating depression also treats suicide. [15]

And in 2014, a study published in *Journal of Affective Disorders* compared 2 different talking therapies – CBT and interpersonal therapy (IPT) – and antidepressants and a placebo, and found that neither of these talking therapies nor medication were more effective than the placebo, when using the BDI-II questionnaire to measure suicidal ideation. That means that neither talking therapy nor antidepressants changed the answer to the question *"Over the last two weeks, how often have you had suicidal thoughts or wishes?"* any more than a placebo. [16]

While this might all sound quite negative, there is a large study with a mainly male group that shows talking therapy *was* effective for men having thoughts about suicide. In 2019, a study published in *Women's Health Issues* followed 1,416 male and 364 female military veterans through a course of talking therapy. [17] This study is rare in that it actually breaks down the difference between women and men, which many studies on talking therapy don't do. They measured the outcomes on thoughts about suicide and found that:

- IPT reduced suicide scores by over 70% in women, and about 55% in men.
- CBT reduced suicide scores by about 65% in women, and about 50% in men.
- Acceptance and commitment therapy (ACT) reduced suicide scores by about 55% in women, and about 40% in men.

So while there were significant improvements for both men and women, all forms of talking therapy tested were less effective for men than women.

The article I referred to earlier highlights the focus of talking therapy is what makes the difference. However, although there are forms of talking therapy that focus on addressing thoughts about suicide, most men who reach out for help don't receive this specific kind of support. [18]

What I want to make crystal clear here is that I'm not discouraging anyone (regardless of gender) from using talking therapy. But it's important that when people are signposted to talking therapies, those talking therapies are relevant for the issues they are experiencing.

For example, UK charity James' Place offers free and in-person therapy for men for men in suicidal crisis in Liverpool, London, and Newcastle. This form of therapy is tailored to address thoughts about suicide, including their "Lay your cards on the Table" intervention, where men stand next to their therapist and lay out a bespoke set of cards that focus on the specific issues that are causing their thoughts about suicide and what they can do about it. The service has been found to reduce distress and entrapment, both risk factors associated with suicide. [19]

In short, it's possible that men reaching out for help to tackle thoughts about suicide are not necessarily being given the most appropriate form of talking therapy.

I have also met many men who reached out for help with thoughts about suicide (not depression) and were prescribed antidepressants. But antidepressants have been found to increase risk of suicide; especially in the first few weeks of use, and especially in young people. A 2023 study examined the risk of suicide in young people after they start taking antidepressant medication. [20] Their findings were summarised by Peter Simmons in an article for *Mad in the UK*:

"For those younger than 25, with no history of suicidal behaviour, taking an antidepressant makes you up to three times more likely to attempt suicide, with that likelihood decreasing as you age. For those 25 or older, taking an

antidepressant doesn't help reduce suicide. Similarly, for those at high risk for suicide, taking an antidepressant doesn't reduce the risk." [21]

A 2019 letter published in *Psychology and Psychotherapy* explained that the way suicide risk is measured in drug trials may obscure the danger. The increased risk of suicidal thoughts caused by antidepressants typically occurs in the first few weeks, but many studies average the risk over the entire trial, which hides this short-term spike. When researchers Michael Hengartner and Martin Plöderl reanalysed the drug trail data using a method focussed on early risk, they found that adults starting antidepressants were 2.5× more likely to attempt suicide than those given a placebo. [22]

Their analysis of the drug trial data suggests that antidepressants directly cause one additional suicide attempt for every 242 adults who start treatment, compared with placebo. Similarly, one additional death from suicide occurs for every 1,303 adults who begin an antidepressant. This is particularly concerning when you consider that 1 in 6 adults in the UK is now taking these medications. [23]

While it's difficult to know whether these calculations are the true representations of the risk, Hengartner and Plöderl were not the first to warn of this issue. A decade earlier, Professor Helena Kraemer of Stanford University wrote an article published in *Statistics in Medicine* warning that a commonly used way of measuring risk in drug trials — known as the "*incidence rate*" or "*events per person-years*" — can be "*at best ambiguous, at worst misleading*". [24]

In 2023, an article by *The Telegraph* pointed out that in a UK survey of 1,500 antidepressant users, 50% had experienced thoughts about suicide *after* starting antidepressants. It also pointed out that the manufacturer of Prozac has paid out over $50 million in compensation for suicides and murders associated with the medication. That's just one brand of antidepressant medication, there are many more. [25]

In 1 UK research project, 7,829 articles were analysed from local newspapers that mentioned a death from suicide and antidepressants. The project found that 40% of deaths from overdose involved antidepressants. And in most cases (55%), the antidepressant was the only drug used to cause death. The study concluded:

"If preventing suicide is a primary reason for prescribing antidepressants, this data set includes several thousand people for whom the drugs clearly did not work. Furthermore, about 1,000 people used the drugs that were supposed to alleviate their depression to kill themselves. [...] Reducing the overprescribing of these relatively ineffective and, for some, lethally dangerous substances is suggested, to reduce suicides." [26]

I'm not suggesting that any of this information is new or unknown to those who read medical articles. The risk of suicide is stated on the box that antidepressants come in and on the patient information leaflet that comes with them. But (in my experience) this information is not being adequately communicated to those who are prescribed antidepressants, or their families. I've met many men who started experiencing thoughts about suicide soon after beginning antidepressants, but were extremely surprised when I suggested that there could be a link.

I shouldn't have been the first one to tell them!

Steve, for example, was told by his prescriber that *"antidepressants can make you feel worse before you feel better."* But for someone who had never experienced thoughts of suicide, this vague understatement meant he didn't realise that suicide risk was being hinted at. In my view, this specific risk should have been explained separately and much more clearly, so he would have known what to look out for.

Thankfully, organisations like The OLLIE Foundation are helping to change this. Their Prescription Safe Plan is a free, simple, user-friendly tool that helps patients and professionals stay alert to mental health side effects from medication. [27] It encourages clear communication and early action. You can download the latest version of the Prescription Safe Plan, available in the 15 most used languages in the UK, from the Resources page on my website. Based on the evidence we've explored, tools like this could save lives.

Not only is there increased risk when you first start taking antidepressants, there is also increased risk when you stop. Studies have shown that the recommended tapering schedules, typically lasting just a few weeks or months, regularly cause severe withdrawal symptoms. These severe symptoms can be mistaken for a return of depression. One study in *The Lancet Psychiatry* found that, to avoid these serious symptoms, patients may need to continue tapering antidepressants for months or even years — and in doses much smaller than those readily available. This is very different from the recommended guidelines. [28]

In 2021, an article published in *Therapeutic Advances in Psychopharmacology* stated that:

"Antidepressant withdrawal is experienced by about half of people who try to reduce or come off their medication. It can be a debilitating, long lasting process. Many clinicians misdiagnose or minimise symptoms, inadvertently prolonging suffering. Most are unable to help patients safely taper off." [29]

The authors found that — with their healthcare provider unable to help — many people are turning to peer support in the form of Facebook groups. The 13 groups they studied were run by ordinary people, not medical practitioners, and had 67,000 members. Over the course of the study (13 months), membership of these groups grew by a staggering 28%. The most common reason for people seeking out the groups was that their healthcare provider hadn't been able to help them to discontinue their antidepressants. The title of the article says it all: *"The role of Facebook groups in the management and raising of awareness of antidepressant withdrawal: is social media filling the void left by health services?"*

I know there are many who have found antidepressants useful and effective, did not experience thoughts about suicide from the medication, and were able to safely come off them when they wanted. So while there may be risks, antidepressants may be a vital form of support for some. My issue with antidepressants is that people who take them are often *not made aware of these risks*.

When men do reach out for help with their mental health, they are often offered talking therapy that does little to reduce suicide, or prescribed antidepressants linked to increased suicide risk. If the help they receive is ineffective or even increases the risk of suicide, getting more men to seek it won't necessarily save more lives.

Christopher attended talking therapy, but it didn't help him to address the reason his work and, consequently, sense of success had dried up. Steve reached out for help with his physical health, and was prescribed medications associated with increased risk of suicide. When he attended the training provided by the NHS, he was taught that he should be aiming for a total cholesterol level of below between 5 and 3.1 mmol/L – which is associated with increased suicide risk in men.

Gary attended peer support groups with other men, but it didn't involve him exploring or addressing his issues with money. When Jaden reached out for help, he was prescribed antidepressants. Three weeks later, his thoughts about suicide started. He had to turn to online peer support when he suffered from withdrawal symptoms and his doctor wasn't able to suggest how to taper them safely.

These are all issues that are buried when people say *"75% of deaths from suicide are men. Despite this, only 36% of referrals to talking therapy are men."*

The reason why this statement seems sound is because it sounds so logical, but it could lead people in the wrong direction, and that's where the real danger lies.

In the words of Dr Paul Quinnett, founder and CEO of the QPR Institute, whose 16,000 active certified QPR instructors have trained more than 5 million people in how to prevent suicide:

"So long as we keep repeating the phrase, 'encourage male help-seeking behavior' in our grant applications, public health marketing, and outreach efforts, suicidal men will just keep dying. Hoping men will become more like women is costing us the lives of our fathers, brothers, sons, uncles, and nephews." [30]

Men are talking; but are we listening?

One of the things that really surprised me when I started learning about male mental health was how little research there actually is into men and suicide. That's not just my opinion, here's an extract from a 2015 article:

"Despite higher rates of suicide in men, there is a [lack] of research examining the perspectives and experiences of males at risk of suicide, particularly in terms of understanding how interventions can be tailored to men's specific needs." [31]

The authors of this statement carried out a study where they interviewed 35 male suicide survivors, and 47 family and friends of male suicide survivors. Amongst other relevant things, the study found that:

"[...] Suicidal ideation may be reduced through provision of practical help to manage crises, and helping men to focus on obligations and their role within families. Findings suggest that interventions for men at risk of suicidal behaviours need to be tailored to specific risk indicators, developmental factors, care needs and individuals' preferences. To our knowledge this is the first qualitative study to explore the experiences of both suicidal men and their family/friends after a suicide attempt, with the view to improve understanding of the processes which are effective in interrupting suicide and better inform interventions for men at risk."

The authors believe that this study was the first to try to understand how to help men who are having thoughts about suicide, and yet it was only published in 2015! It's also very small, but I'll take a small study over no study at all.

And what is already known about mental health is often unhelpful when it comes to supporting men, because it combines findings for men and women. This leaves no understanding of their unique challenges and perspectives. To quote Samaritans:

"In general, studies of interventions to reduce suicide fail to report on the demographic details of their participants and tend to combine outcomes for participants from different gender, ethnic or socioeconomic groups; and there are few studies evaluating interventions developed explicitly for 'high risk' demographic groups [like men]." [32]

In 2014, an article published in *Frontiers in Neuroendocrinology* stated that some of the significant sex differences in mental health may be explained by hormonal differences. Women are twice as likely to suffer from depression and anxiety than men, and are most vulnerable around periods of hormonal change. Men, on the other hand, have higher levels of testosterone - a hormone found to protect against depression in men, women, and animals. [33]

But there is another side to hormonal differences. Research has found that the amount of testosterone children are exposed to in the womb ("prenatal testosterone") influences how their brains develop. For example, higher levels of prenatal testosterone are linked to lower empathy and less eye contact, but stronger skills in systematic thinking, in both boys and girls aged 6–9. [34] [35]

The amount of testosterone a male received in the womb also leaves a clue on his hands. Men who received a higher dose of prenatal testosterone while they were developing in the womb are thought to have a slightly longer ring finger than their index finger. Males who receive lower levels of testosterone in the womb are thought to have shorter ring fingers. The difference is very minor, but it stays the same for the rest of a man's life. This ratio between these 2 fingers is known as the "2D:4D ratio". Testosterone levels in the womb and the 2D:4D ratio have been found to be associated with:

"[..] Numerical competencies, spatial skills, handedness, cognitive abilities, academic performance, sperm counts, personalities and prevalence of obesity, migraine, eating disorders, depression, myopia, autism." [36]

Plus some less serious things. In one study, a panel of 104 female judges watched videos of men dancing and then rated them based on their attractiveness. Men with the most masculinised 2D:4D ratios were rated significantly higher on attractiveness than men with a more feminised 2D:4D ratio. [37]

Why is this relevant in a book about male mental health?

In 2019, a report published in *Progress in Neurobiology* compared the 2D:4D ratios of men who had survived a suicide attempt, with those who had died from suicide. They found that men who survived a suicide attempt had a less masculinised 2D:4D ratio - indicating a less masculinised brain organisation. The men who died from suicide had a more masculinised 2D:4D ratio, indicting a more masculinised brain organisation. It appears that brain biology could play a role in male suicide attempts being more lethal. [38]

We've just explored some studies that offer a potential biological explanation for why:

- Men are less likely to suffer from depression and anxiety, but
- Men are more likely to die from their suicide attempts.

And yet, I never see any of these biological findings referenced in conversations around male mental health or suicide prevention. Instead, we often hear that men are dying from suicide because *"they don't reach out for help"*.

I don't think we should shy away from exploring these biological differences. Just because something is biological, doesn't mean it is destiny. If anything, the opposite is true. Once we understand something in more detail, we have a better chance of changing it.

But rather than study men to understand what they need when it comes to suicide, rather than try to understand why generic support might not be working for men, and rather than investigate these biological factors, we often blame men. In the words of an article published in the *Journal of Adolescent Health*:

"Adolescent boys and young adult men have been identified as a neglected group within health policy and intervention domains. They have also been somewhat blamed for their relatively poor help-seeking attitudes and behaviors rather than being proactively engaged by systems that are purposively designed to assist them." [39]

In *Invisible Women: Exposing Data Bias in a World Designed for Men*, Caroline Criado Perez reveals how a widespread gender data gap results in systems, products, and policies that often ignore or disadvantage women. From car safety tests and medical research to public transport planning and personal protective equipment (PPE), the book shows how defaulting to male data leads to real-world consequences for women's health, safety, and wellbeing. [40]

Is it possible, then, that the same thing could have happened the other way around when it comes to mental health? I think it is. It seems to me that even well intentioned research is based on what works for women. So when another man dies by suicide, people will assume that he didn't reach out for help, even though he may have. "*What a shame,*" some people will say, "*that men don't feel able to reach out for help.*"

The world is waking up to the fact that women shouldn't be treated like small men. And yet we still treat men as if they're women who don't talk about how they feel.

So far in this section, I have been focussing on why the current approach may not be working for men. My aim is not to discourage anyone from reaching out for help, but to encourage us to look deeper than the fallacy that men are "*not reaching out for help.*" The reality is that when men do reach out, thoughts about suicide are often conflated with depression, and medications are sometimes prescribed that can actually increase suicide risk. When men attend talking therapies, the focus is often on addressing depression, not the factors most closely associated with suicide in men. In short, the support available might not be targeting the underlying causes. This doesn't mean men shouldn't use the support that's available, but it does suggest there is an opportunity to save lives by offering services that are more relevant and effective for men who are at risk of suicide.

I believe that to truly support men, we need to recognise that talking is only the first step — not the solution. Next, men need to know what to talk about and what changes to make. One of the most direct ways to do this is to help men to connect with what matters most: their purpose.

How masculinity impacts male mental health

I was 15 years old when I had my last full day of school.

One Friday afternoon, I was taking my seat in class, and our teacher was out of the room. A boy called Jamie walked in, and began acting intimidatingly towards some of my classmates. Jamie was known for causing trouble in school – and filming it – especially when teachers weren't around. I knew immediately it was a bad situation, but I didn't realise that the next 5 minutes would change the trajectory of my life.

(As elsewhere in this book, names and identifying details have been changed to protect privacy. This story reflects my experience and is not meant to cast anyone in a negative light. It happened a long time ago, and people can change—I know I have.)

Standing at the back of the classroom, Jamie towered over a boy called Richard, who sat in fear looking up at Jamie's phone camera lens. The room was silent – a rare thing in a boys' school – and tense. Nobody wanted Jamie to hit Richard, but at the same time, nobody wanted to distract Jamie and become the new target. The tension grew, and I knew Richard was about to be attacked. Then I did something and surprised myself.

I slid my books into my bag, stood up, took off my glasses and said, "Leave him alone, Jamie."

It seemed to take about 5 minutes for Jamie to turn his head to me and smile. In reality, it was probably only a second. His phone followed his gaze. He slowly moved towards me like an armoured tank approaching a lonely soldier; his arm extended at me like a turret, until the camera was just 6 inches from my face. I looked into the lens and wished for the teacher to return to the room.

"Who *the fuck* are you?" he demanded.

Then... Whack! His right palm hit me across the face. I stumbled 2 steps backwards, then straightened myself back up again. There was no way I was going to fight back. I could take a slap, but I didn't want Jamie to jump over the table and strangle me. I would comply.

As I opened my mouth to reason with him, he drew his right hand back again – this time behind his head –and hit me twice as hard. I held on to my desk, to avoid falling back into my chair. Other than his hand hitting my face, the room was silent.

I looked up, into Jamie's face. My cheek was swelling, my ears ringing. I could tell a third strike was coming. This time, he drew his hand back so far that I was confident he was going to knock me over. His hand flew towards me... Then stopped an inch from my face. He flicked my stinging cheek with his forefinger. Then chuckled like he had heard a weak joke.

As he put away his phone, my teacher entered the room. She told Jamie to leave, because he wasn't in this class. "Sit down, Ryan," she said as she turned her back to me and began writing the date on the whiteboard.

I picked up my bag and headed to the deputy headmaster's office. I wanted them to know that Jamie was randomly assaulting students, who were just trying to learn. But when the deputy head learned what happened, he seemed more interested in Jamie than anyone else.

"Did he hit the teacher, Ryan? That's something we've been worried about." When I explained that Jamie didn't hit the teacher, the door was closed in my face. I heard the deputy head on the phone, asking Jamie to return to school. "You're not necessarily in trouble, Jamie," I heard him say. "We just want to check you're safe." No students were allowed phones in school, and yet my deputy head seemed to have Jamie's mobile number? The situation was getting more unfair by the minute.

So there I was, standing in the hallway outside of the deputy head's office. My face swelling and my ear ringing. While my deputy head assured Jamie that he wasn't in trouble. And I stood alone in a corridor, waiting for Jamie to return...

Waiting to see what he would do when he found out that I had run to a teacher.

I had to get out of the school.

That's when I walked out of the school's back gate. For me, secondary school was over.

Then began some of the darkest months of my life. I was stuck at home, with no skills, no job, no money, and no girlfriend. No structure, nothing to do, and no reason to get out of bed in the morning. I became very depressed. I slept all day and spent all night on the internet. The only thing that motivated me was spending the nights learning about anything to do with mechanics. I studied car engines, guns, and how planes stay in the sky. Besides that, I didn't do much else and I didn't want to leave the house.

But through a friend, I got the opportunity to do a week's work experience at a local gunsmith – a workshop where they repaired the shotguns used for clay pigeon shooting competitions and pheasant hunting. That was the only interest I had at the time, the only thing that would motivate me.

During the week's work experience, I found that I could contribute to the team, even though I wasn't yet a good engineer. Just a simple task like making tea or taking the guns to be test-fired saved others time and made me feel... Useful.

At the end of the work experience week, I was given my first job offer, along with some cash in exchange for my time. I wasn't expecting it, but I knew exactly what I was going to do with the money.

That Friday afternoon, as I rode my bike home, I tore through the shallow rivers – rather than take the bridges – to save time. When I arrived back at home, dripping in river water and sweat, I handed all the cash to my mum to help her to pay the rent.

This was the turning point in my life.

I had gone from having no structure, to having a whole team around me. From having no reason to get up, to needing to be somewhere, else I would let others down. From feeling **like a burden**, to feeling *useful*.

I worked as a gunsmith until I was 19. For the first 2 years, I used to cycle every day on my bike with my toolkit on my back. I cycled through the summer sun, the winter snow, and the rain. By today's standards, the workshop was dirty and dangerous. We worked every day with unpleasant chemicals that stained our skin, but we were all too macho to wear any gloves. The machines didn't have the kind of guards you would expect, and so it would have been easy to have an accident.

During the winter, the workshop was so cold I could see my breath in front of me. Sometimes my hands were too cold to grip my tools, so I would go next door and make tea for everyone, as a way of warming up.

The kitchen was warmer as it was in the same room where toxic chemicals were heated up to 350°C to turn the guns black. The fumes really didn't have anywhere to go, which meant we breathed them in while we did the washing up. Once they saw the conditions, most clients turned down the offer of a cup of tea.

But this dirty, dangerous, cold job gave me meaning in my life. An intrinsic part of the job was learning that when something is broken, you don't just repair the damage, you also have to identify the root cause to prevent it happening again. Something that stayed with me.

At age 19, I left engineering to learn how to be a better communicator and business person. The way I did this was by working in small organisations and finding role models within those businesses. At age 23, a former boss offered me a role co-founding a business with him. He was one of my role models at the time, and so it was a dream job. I went on to grow the business and our team. The work was always challenging, but I was good at it. It gave me an enormous sense of purpose, and I took pride in hiring, training and coaching young people, which was not common in our industry. This was the business I was working in when I heard about Brad.

For six years, I worked most evenings and weekends. I bought an apartment and always drove nice cars. But beneath the surface, things in the company were shifting in ways I didn't fully understand at the time. After a series of negotiations, my equity changed, and the balance of power within the board shifted. Eventually, I realised my role was shrinking, my decisions ignored, and my sense of belonging gone. I was no longer part of the company's future.

At age 29, I had to walk away from the business that had been my source of purpose for 6 years. This meant walking away from the team I had hired, trained and been a part of. I felt I had failed them — failed to see the politics unfolding around me, and failed to protect what I had built.

It felt just like when I had walked out of school. I had no job and no team. No structure, nothing to do, and no reason to get out of bed in the morning... I knew I had to act *fast*.

The first step was to secure another job, even if that meant only covering my bills. That would take care of Protecting the Cave, and give me a sense of security. Then I would do some coaching work to share what I had learned about male mental health with other men. This would make me feel useful again, if my new role didn't. I knew what I needed to do.

I wanted to share this story with you because in the 2 darkest moments of my life – despite how depressed or stressed I was – I didn't want to reach out for professional help with my own mental health.

Looking back, I think there were 3 main reasons for this. During these personal moments of crisis:

1. My problem was that I didn't feel useful.
2. Having used talking therapy in the past, I didn't personally believe it would help with this challenge.
3. I didn't want to deprive anyone else of support who needed it more.

I know now that I wasn't alone. In 2023, a study of 725 men who had recently experienced thoughts about suicide asked these men whether they had reached out for help, and - if not - why not? The most common reason men in the study gave for not reaching out for help was that they did not believe that support would help (43%). Only 16% of the men said that they didn't reach out for help because of the social costs (stigma, embarrassment). Of those who didn't believe support would be effective, their main reason for thinking this was that **they had reached out for help in the past, and had a bad experience**. The results were published in *Current Psychology* and showed: [41]

"Participant responses revealed a range of negative encounters. Most men appeared to find previous help to be pointless, unhelpful, and ineffective. For a smaller group, therapy offered temporary relief, but was not beneficial over the long term. Other men suggested that the support they received amplified their feelings of suicide."

During the personal challenges I had, I did not have any thoughts about suicide. But I understand what the men in this study were saying. The support available just wasn't what they needed at the time.

In 2020, Samaritans interviewed men who had reached out for support in the past and asked them what makes an engaging support service. They found that:

"*The opportunity to make a contribution, a feeling of inclusivity and the opportunity to work towards common goals were key facets of an engaging service, according to those we spoke to.*"

"*The men with lived experience who took part in our research were clear about what could be done to engage and support them more effectively, and what had worked for them in the past. All services should apply this lived insight throughout the development and delivery of their services.*"

"*Rather than framing services around help-seeking, which can imply that there is something 'wrong' with men, services and initiatives should consider how men could be given opportunities to contribute. This could involve co-running or facilitating the service as well as just attending.*" [42]

It seems to me that these men are saying they want an opportunity to feel useful. Just as I did when I crashed out of school and left the job I loved.

Back in Part 2: Achieving Recognition, I shared a small study that found the best way for men to overcome thoughts about suicide is to take steps towards being their ideal self. That study also found that men needed to feel needed by others. [43]

And in 2017, a study published in *Personality and Social Psychology Bulletin* followed a group of people (women and men) who took part in a peer support group online. They found that supporting others improved the mental health of participants more than receiving support, and more than talking about their own problems. [44]

This absolutely reflects my own experience that supporting others has often been better for me than receiving support. Of course, there were times when I needed support too. I have always reached out for help when I have needed it, but it's been practical help. I reached out for things like skills to help me to find a new job, to talk to strangers, to improve my public speaking. I am very pro-support and pro reaching out for help, but I want practical help that leads to me being more useful. I don't appear to be alone here either. When I started completing the Future Call exercise with men, I found that their most aspirational goals were often based around giving back and being useful to others. These conversations became the foundations of what became Able to Serve.

One way I build this knowledge into my coaching work is to always ask my clients to hold me - and the other men on my Programme - accountable. Many men have told me that this group accountability was the part that made the biggest difference to them. I wasn't acting like a "guru" with all the answers. I was making them feel useful by giving them something meaningful to do.

But there was another reason I didn't want to reach out for professional support. It was the messaging around men and mental health. Firstly, every article about men and mental health showed photos of men with their heads in their hands, or in floods of tears. Formal support clearly wasn't designed to make you feel useful, it was designed to get you to "open up" and to be "vulnerable".

The way I saw it, I couldn't be useful if I was vulnerable. In fact, I would be the opposite of useful – I would be a burden! And by reaching out for help, I would also be depriving *that man* in the photo from the support he needs. And he clearly needs it more than me. It was the images of men with their head in their hands, tears streaming down their face that made me think that formal support wasn't for me.

This suspicion was verified whenever I read articles about men and mental health, they often stated that *masculinity* itself is a problem that puts men at risk. I always had a sense that, if I was to accept help, I would have to accept that masculinity is "bad". But I wasn't prepared to do that. To me, masculinity meant being useful, being a team player, and being able to provide. None of these were values I was prepared to give up. And so reaching out for formal support was not an option to me.

Again, this isn't unique to me. Studies that interview men about what masculinity means to them find that there isn't a universal definition of masculinity. To some, masculinity is about creativity, sensitivity, and intelligence. Are these harmful values? I don't think so. [45]

So if masculinity means different things to different men, how can anyone say whether it is "bad" or "good"?

I think it comes down to a stereotypical image of masculinity, which is often called "*hegemonic masculinity*". "Hegemonic" means dominant, and hegemonic masculinity is the idea that a "real man" is one that is not feminine, and is able to compete against and dominate others. This ideal is believed to make men less likely to reach out for help when they need it. And it is this form of masculinity that has probably led to masculinity being blamed for men having worse mental and physical health outcomes. On stages, on panels and in private conversations, I am often asked: "*It's because of masculinity, right?*" [46] [47]

But even hegemonic masculinity – often described as a problem – appears to have its benefits when it comes to engaging men in conversations around mental health. In a small study published in 2006, researchers interviewed men about masculinity and depression, and found that:

"*Very little research exists which examines men's experiences of depression. [...] We found that, as part of recovery from depression, it was important for men to reconstruct a valued sense of themselves and their own masculinity. The most common strategy was to incorporate values associated with hegemonic masculinity into narratives (being 'one of the boys', re-establishing control, and responsibility to others). [...] Generalisations about depressed men always being silent are misleading.*" [48]

Paradoxically, traditionally masculine values could be a hook used to engage men in conversations about mental health. I definitely agree with that.

It is true that studies have found elements of traditional (hegemonic) masculinity that are associated with increased risk – specifically *self-reliance* and *risk-taking*. But to keep things in context, a study of Australian construction workers found that neither of these two traits were associated with suicide as much as *work-related stresses* (high work demand, low job control, or lack of role clarity). So maybe we should focus on that first, before blaming a person's gender identity? [49]

I can't say this better than Andy Cook, chief executive at the UK's Centre for Social Justice:

"We must stop seeing masculinity as a problem to be solved and start seeing it as a strength to be nurtured. Strength, resilience, responsibility – these are not traits to be suppressed but harnessed for good." [50]

The criticisms of masculinity certainly made me feel that formal support was not for men like me. It wasn't for men who believed that masculinity could be a good thing. In 2012, Samaritans picked up on this, and recommended that:

"[...] A new 'face' is put on suicide prevention for men, with suicide prevention measures understanding what it is 'to be a man' and the availability of more men to talk to. [...] Interventions need to engage and work with 'who men are' and what is important to them at this time." [51]

I think that criticising masculinity is a mistake, as by doing so, we inadvertently miss out on one of the easiest ways to engage men in a conversation about mental health: by linking it to strength. Mental health support should be "sold" to men as a way to be stronger, more successful, and more useful. After all, that's how almost everything else is successfully marketed to men.

But for all the reasons to believe that masculinity could be positive when it comes to mental health, there is one aspect of masculinity that I believe can be as harmful as it is helpful. Something that requires and deserves a detailed understanding.

Heroic sacrifice.

When life lacks purpose, death feels meaningful

When I first read Franz de Waal's book *Different: What Apes Can Teach Us About Gender* there was a section that I just couldn't forget:

"Since male gorillas are hyper protective, Western hunters in the old days usually brought back the skins, heads, and hands of adult males. Males bluff-charged

the hunters so as to give their family time to escape, and they were shot. Nowadays, thankfully, the same defensive actions result in lots of pictures of imposing chest-beating males." [52]

This image really stuck with me, and I couldn't help but talk about it during coaching calls with men. When I told Jaden about it, he said, "You know, when you told me that story about the gorilla, the hair on my arms stood on end. I had a lump in my throat. I couldn't help but think what a *masculine act* it was for that gorilla to sacrifice himself for his family."

And that's when something hit me. If there's one thing that can instantly elevate any man (or gorilla!) to being a hero, it is sacrifice. Once I was alerted to it, I realised it was a common theme shared between fictional and real male heroes.

For decades, James Bond was a polarising figure. While seen by some as an action hero, others see Bond as a chauvinistic and womanising anti-hero. In the last movie in the Daniel Craig saga (*No Time to Die*), Bond fights his way through many "bad guys", kills his main enemy, and essentially saves the whole world. But, on finding out that he is carrying a virus that will kill his daughter if he leaves the bad guy's lair, he stands on the roof of a bunker under a missile strike from the Royal Navy, ending his life. Before the missiles rain down, we see Bond standing on the roof, looking up. Next to the blood leaking into his shirt, his daughter's soft toy bunny tucked under his braces. He dies a hero.

Another character who comes up a lot in conversations with men (and boys) is Maximus Decimus Meridius, the main character in the movie *Gladiator*. When Maximus' wife and son are abused and murdered, he fights his way to their revenge. But after finally killing Commodus (the emperor who ordered the execution of his family) Maximus dies in the Coliseum. Through his sacrifice, he dies a hero.

In the 1996 film *Independence Day*, Robert Casse is a retired combat fighter pilot whose stories of being abducted by aliens are ignored. His son thinks Robert is a loser. When the aliens arrive, as Casse predicted, humanity is in a fight for survival. In the climax of the film, Casse finds himself in a fighter jet, trying to fire a missile at the alien mothership. He has a chance to destroy it, but the missile won't detach from his fighter jet. Does Casse turn his fighter jet around? No. He shouts the legendary words "Hello, boys. I'm baaaaaaaack!" as he flies his jet into the mothership, setting off the missile, saving the world, and killing himself in the process. In the control room, a man turns to Casse's son who watched his dad's last act on a screen. "What your father did was very brave. You should be extremely proud." Casse's death took him from being labelled by others as a loser, to becoming the hero of the film. Most importantly, a hero in his son's eyes.

I grew up playing video games and my personal hero was a character in Hideo Kojima's *Metal Gear Solid*. His codename was Solid Snake. Snake was always on a one-way mission into the enemy territory. He had to destroy the bad guy and save the world. How we would get out after infiltrating the base was an afterthought. First, the mission had to be accomplished. There was something about this heroic sacrifice that made me want to be him.

This idyllic image of heroic sacrifice isn't solely found in fiction, but is a constant theme surrounding real war heroes. The "Charge of the Light Brigade," a 19th-century British military mishap, saw cavalrymen ordered to ride into a valley of near-certain death, surrounded by enemy artillery. They were later hailed as heroes for following orders despite knowing there would be heavy losses. The British poet Tennyson even wrote a poem about the charge, urging us to honour their '*glory*'. More than a century later, during World War I, British recruitment campaigns portrayed army enlistment as a noble and heroic act, and around 2.67 million young men volunteered over the course of the war - almost as many as the 2.77 million who were conscripted. I've also known several men to describe the US Paratroopers in the 101st Airborne Division (F Company, 327th Glider Infantry Regiment) as their role models. In World War II, when outnumbered, surrounded, short on supplies and given the choice to surrender or be annihilated, this group of paratroopers defiantly sent their German enemies the simple message: "*NUTS!*" The threat of death did not deter them from their job of holding their position. What seems to make men like these heroes in the eyes of other men is their heroic sacrifice to complete their missions. [53][54][55]

And when I see boys playing in the park or at a family party, I often see the same thing. The dramatic clutching of the chest, falling to the ground, struggling, and then drawing their last breath. They are pretending to die. The heroic death, reserved for the most heroic characters.

To me, the underlying message from these characters, traditions, and games is the same: men will be remembered as a hero, if they'll only be willing to die for a good cause. This act of sacrifice is the ultimate way for men to prove they are both capable and moral. It's what makes men heroes in the eyes of other men.

Before we start blaming movies, books, or army recruitment campaigns for 'brainwashing' men into believing that sacrifice is meaningful, it's worth remembering that male gorillas do it too — suggesting this drive might be more ingrained than societal conditioning. I believe that stories of heroic sacrifice resonate with men and boys because they appeal to something felt by all of us: the need to find purpose and meaning. I'm not suggesting that the search for meaning — or the willingness to sacrifice oneself for others — is uniquely male. But men often see physical risk, even the possibility of death, as a way to be useful to others.

In January 2025, after a week of working together, I talked through this very idea with George Peterkin over dinner. George is a psychotherapist, ex-teacher in a boys' school, and an eating disorder therapist. He shared with me how he was once working with a man who was continuously talking about a heroic death. But the turning point in their work together came when George asked the question, "*What would a heroic life look like?*"

I believe this concept of heroic sacrifice shows up in everyday life, shaping men's choices and behaviours in ways that are often invisible at first. This can include men not taking time off work, not looking after their own wellbeing, or not reaching out for help when it's needed. I also believe it's the reason that I felt compelled to stand up to Jamie, when it looked like he was going to hurt Richard.

In a study of 1,000 men, it was found that 40% wouldn't reach out for help with their mental health. Of those who wouldn't reach out, the main reason was that they had learned to deal with it themselves (40%), followed by the fact they **didn't want to be a burden to anyone else**. Only 29% mentioned embarrassment, while 20% mentioned stigma. [56]

I believe that when life lacks purpose, death can feel meaningful to men. That's why the only sustainable way to tackle male suicide is to give men the tools they need to **find a reason to live**. A way to be useful. A purpose that makes the pain, risk, and discomfort of life worth it.

Most importantly, this is not a cheap trick to convince men to live. The reason I believe it worked for George's client, and the reason it worked for Jaden, is because life really is purposeful. But only when we use what we have right now to make a difference to others.

Able to Serve: Strategies

Able to Serve is about a man's sense of purpose. In this part of the book, we have explored how lack of purpose impacts mental health in men, and the protective role of feeling useful. We can support the men we care about by helping them to identify ways to use their skills and strengths to support others.

❏ Identify skills and strengths

I'm going to share with you a structured coaching exercise that has been helpful for many men, and also for me. In theory, this could work as part of a casual conversation, but I find it's more effective to follow a structured process. You'll need a pen, paper, and an environment free of distractions.

You say: "Ryan's got this exercise that men have used to find more purpose and meaning in life. It takes about five minutes and some thinking, but it can be useful. Often the best things come to mind once the exercise is completed. Do you want to try it and see if it's useful for you?"

Assuming it's a "yes", next you say: "I'm going to set a timer for sixty seconds, and you have to write down your strengths and skills. You can write down anything. Be honest; not modest. It doesn't matter whether you enjoy doing these things or not, the question is 'are you good at them?' You do not have to share the list with me or with anyone else, unless you want to. This list is for your own use only. Ready? Go."

Neither of you should talk during the 60-second timer. If he looks like he has run out of things to write, wait for the full 60 seconds to be up. If he is still writing at the end of the timer, just let him finish. I've found it's important to not pay any attention to the list yourself. If you're with him in person, don't even look at it. This is a self-discovery exercise, rather than a sharing exercise.

One of the things I really like about this exercise is that being "instructed" to write a list of things you're good at is like being forced to accept how capable you are. You'll see in the last part of this book that helping men to feel capable is a big part of what we're trying to achieve when we support them.

"OK, next we're going to do the same thing, but this time you're going to write a separate list of the things you enjoy doing. Some things might be the same as the previous list, but some might be different. You're allowed to write anything you like in the sixty seconds, and you don't have to show me or anybody the list. Ready? Go."

Once the 2 initial lists are complete, you can say:

"I want you to label the first list (strengths and skills) 'A'. Now label the second list (things you like doing) 'B'."

Now we can move on to the next step.

❏ Serve people / causes that matter most

More lists…!

"Next, I'm going to set a timer for sixty seconds and I want you to write down the names of the people you care the most about. Go."

Once that is complete:

"This time I'm going to set another timer, and I want you to write down a list of causes you believe in. They might be organisations, or a more general issue that needs to be addressed in the world. Again, sixty seconds…"

It's quite typical that the lists get shorter as the exercise progresses. When it comes to the 'causes you believe in' list, men often write nothing for the first 50 seconds. But this thinking time is extremely valuable. It is a gift to be given the time and space to just think about what matters to you in life. If he says "That's hard", just smile and nod your head. Something will come. Once the third and fourth lists are complete, you can say:

"You can probably guess what I am about to say. Label the list of important people 'C' and the list of causes you believe in 'D'."

Now he has these 4 lists that you probably haven't seen, it's time to bring this all together.

❏ Support family, friends, and faith

"You're going to do more writing now to bring this all together. I'm going to give you a sentence that you are going to write down and finish: 'Some ways I could use A (my strengths and skills) to benefit C and D would be to…' I'm going to set a timer for sixty seconds. Write down as many things as you can think of."

The timer will be counting down for 60 seconds, but if he is still writing at the end of the timer, just let him keep going. Like before, don't look or pry to see what's been written down. Now there's another step:

"Next, finish this sentence: 'Some ways I could use B (things I like doing) to benefit C and D would be to…' Sixty seconds. Go."

I like this exercise because it is all about using what you have right now to support the people and causes you believe in. That is what it takes to feel useful. I also like the fact that I (as coach) do not need to see what people have written down. It gives a sense of autonomy to the person completing the exercise. Not sharing the list allows him to write whatever comes to mind without fear of judgement or embarrassment.

Lots of sources of purpose and meaning have come out of this exercise. After completing this exercise, Christopher decided to hire his dad as his executive assistant. This gave his dad a way to feel useful and (although it cost Christopher a little income) meant that they could spend quality time together.

When Steve completed this exercise, he decided to set Saturday afternoon aside each week to clean and maintain his daughter's car. As a former mechanic, it was extremely satisfying for him to use those skills once again, and he enjoyed helping his daughter hang on to more of her money. But it was something that he didn't realise would be meaningful, until he completed this exercise.

This exercise helped me realise I should donate all of the money I am paid for coaching to good causes. It took me months to put it into action, but once I had written those words, I couldn't stop thinking about it. (However, my talks and training do make a profit for me and my family – can't forget Protecting the Cave!)

This step in The ALPHA Framework is called 'Support your friends, family, and faith' because they are ways that many men have found meaning in life, but following the exercise in this section can allow men to go deeper and make powerful connections.

Actually, there is also a final question you can add to this exercise that can be life-changing:

"Lastly, complete this sentence: 'Something that scares me but would change my life forever would be to...'"

In response to this, Jaden wrote: "Something that scares me but would change my life forever would be to get over my fear of having money, get a qualification in money management, and create a trust fund for Amiee."

Two years before writing this book, I wrote: "Something that scares me but would change my life forever would be to have a baby with Emma." I am now a dad.

And about a year ago, this exercise prompted me to tackle my self-doubt head on and publish a book, because it might actually help someone.

❏ Be part of a team

For all the reasons we've explored, teamwork is extremely important for male mental health. It can be difficult for us to feel like part of a team in the modern world. With flexible and remote working becoming more normal, we're less likely to connect with others at work.

When I work with emergency service providers, they often tell me that when they joined the job decades ago, your "shift" or "watch" was like your family. You knew what each other were going through and you would support one another. You would be together while you worked and then together afterwards for a "debrief" in the bar (oh, how times have changed). But now rotas are more changeable, and you are partnered up with different people each time you go out. While this gives organisations more operational flexibility, it means frontline responders may have lost the sense of teamwork that once protected them from the stress of the role.

When I work with men in the construction industry, they tell me that the fractured nature of the industry means it's sometimes hard to tell who is on your team. Men who work in offices tell me that flexible and remote working – while beneficial in many ways – often leave them feeling without a sense of team.

The workplace isn't the only place men can find a sense of teamwork. I learned years ago to ask men who recently started feeling down, "Have you recently left a team?" I was surprised how often they told me that they had recently left a 5-a-side football team, a hockey team, or a bridge team. A good team gives everyone the opportunity to use what they have to serve one another, and a wider purpose.

❏ Say "no" to unfulfilling things

Sometimes, living a more meaningful life comes down to nothing more than simply saying "no" to the things we don't find meaningful. This frees up time for the things that matter.

I've learned from coaching that Purpose = Values + Action.

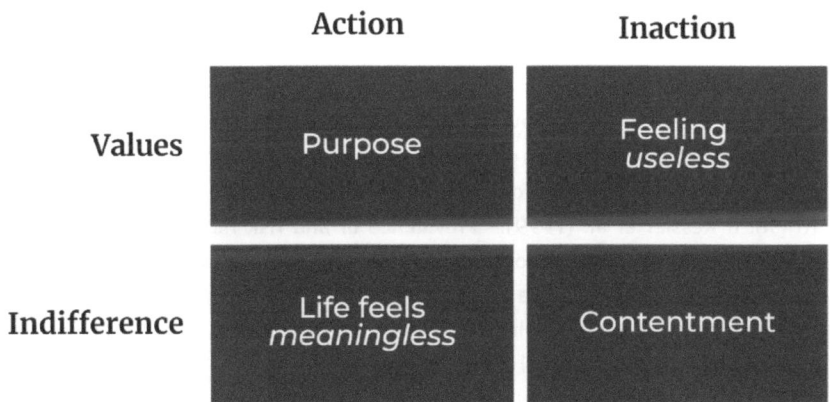

When men have values but don't commit any action to those values, they can start to feel useless. Of course, nobody is useless, this is just a trick our brain plays on us from time to time. Similarly, when men are busy taking action but not on things they value, they can start to feel that life is meaningless. Sometimes, these 2 sensations occur at the same time.

Both action and inaction are fundamental to the notion of purpose. When men take **action on their values**, that leads to a **feeling of purpose**. And when men **don't take action** on things they are **indifferent** about, it can lead to a feeling of **contentment**.

To help men who are "busy" doing things that they are indifferent about, you can ask them to complete this sentence: "My life would be more meaningful if I stopped…"

These answers are more than lightbulb moments. Sometimes they are life-changing.

Ultimately, our aim is to help men identify where their skills and strengths can make a difference, to feel useful by serving causes they believe in, and—where necessary—to show that their life can be more meaningful than their death. These five strategies are ways I believe men can gain a true sense of purpose in life.

ENDNOTES

1. Any study I use as a source won't show the full picture. But if you spend time researching this, you'll see that women have higher suicide attempt rates than men across diverse populations, maintaining this difference even after controlling for age, socioeconomic status, and mental health history. I'll include 3 such articles...
2. R1458: R Kessler et al. (1999). "Prevalence of and risk factors for lifetime suicide attempts in the National Comorbidity Survey." Arch Gen Psychiatry.
3. R1457: A Miranda-Mendizaba et al. (2019). "Gender differences in suicidal behavior in adolescents and young adults: systematic review and meta-analysis of longitudinal studies." International Journal of Public Health.
4. R819: L Lu et al. (2020). "Gender difference in suicidal ideation and related factors among rural elderly: a cross-sectional study in Shandong, China." Annals of General Psychiatry.
5. I'm not going to share a source for this one - there is plenty of evidence out there that you'll find on sites like PubMed. I'd rather not share sources on methods in case it relates to the personal experiences of readers.
6. R195: Mental Health Foundation (2020). "Men and women: Statistics." mentalhealth.org.
7. R146: British Association for Counselling and Psychotherapy (2022). "Men's Health Week: Changing attitudes to mental health and therapy." bacp.co.uk.
8. R1023: Office For National Statistics (2024). "Suicides in England and Wales: 2022 registrations." ons.gov.uk.
9. R158: Samaritans (2012). "Men, suicide and society: Why disadvantaged men in midlife die by suicide" samaritans.org.
10. R672: National Confidential Inquiry into Suicide and Safety in Mental Health (2021). "Suicide by middle-aged men." University of Manchester.
11. R686: Second Step (2023). "Hope project." second-step.co.uk.
12. R158: Samaritans (2012). "Men, suicide and society: Why disadvantaged men in midlife die by suicide." samaritans.org.
13. R298: J S van Bentum et al. (2021). "Cognitive therapy and interpersonal psychotherapy reduce suicidal ideation independent from their effect on depression." Depression and Anxiety.
14. R295: P Cuijpers et al. (2013). "The effects of psychotherapy for adult depression on suicidality and hopelessness: A systematic review and meta-analysis." Journal of Affective Disorders.
15. R300: Sudak & Rajalakshmi (2018). "Reducing suicide risk: The role of psychotherapy." Psychiatric Times.
16. R297: E Weitz et al. (2014). "Do depression treatments reduce suicidal ideation? The effects of CBT, IPT, pharmacotherapy, and placebo on suicidality." Journal of Affective Disorders.
17. R293: M Kumpula et al. (2019). "An evaluation of the effectiveness of evidence-based psychotherapies for depression to reduce suicidal ideation among male and female veterans." Women's Health Issues.

18 R298: J S van Bentum et al (2021). "Cognitive therapy and interpersonal psychotherapy reduce suicidal ideation independent from their effect on depression." Depression and Anxiety.
19 R1517: P Saini et al. (2014). "James' place service evaluation: Year Four Report." Liverpool John Moore's University.
20 R540: T Lagerberg et al. (2023). "Effect of selective serotonin reuptake inhibitor treatment following diagnosis of depression on suicidal behaviour risk: A target trial emulation." Neuropsychopharmacology.
21 R1461: P Simmons (2023). "Antidepressants increase suicide attempts in youth; no preventative effect." Mad in the UK.
22 R452: M P Hengartner et al. (2019). "Newer-generation antidepressants and suicide risk in randomized controlled trials: A re-analysis of the FDA database." Psychotherapy Psychosomatics.
23 R981: S Knapton (2023). 'Antidepressants increase the risk of suicide for some patients, scientists warn.' The Telegraph.
24 R1510: H Kraemer (2009). "Events per person-time (incidence rate): A misleading statistic?" Statistics in Medicine.
25 R981: S Knapton (2023). "Antidepressants increase the risk of suicide for some patients, scientists warn." The Telegraph.
26 R454: J Read (2023). "Antidepressants and suicide: 7,829 inquests in England and Wales, 2003–2020." Ethical Human Psychology and Psychiatry.
27 R499: D Roberts (2023). "Prescription Safe Plan." theolliefoundation.org.
28 R331: M A Horowitz et al. (2019). "Tapering of SSRI treatment to mitigate withdrawal symptoms." The Lancet Psychiatry.
29 R332: E White et al. (2021). "The role of Facebook groups in the management and raising of awareness of antidepressant withdrawal: is social media filling the void left by health services?" Therapeutic Advances in Psychopharmacology.
30 R438: M Pittaro (2021). "Understanding the men who die by suicide." Psychology Today.
31 R170: M Player et al. (2015). "What interrupts suicide attempts in men: A qualitative study." PLOS One.
32 R158: Samaritans (2012). "Men, suicide and society: Why disadvantaged men in midlife die by suicide." samaritans.org.
33 R741: J McHenry et al. (2014). "Sex differences in anxiety and depression: Role of testosterone." Frontiers in Neuroendocrinology.
34 R1467: B Auyeung et al. (2006). "Foetal testosterone and the child systemizing quotient." European Journal of Endocrinology.
35 R1468: E Chapman et al. (2006). "Fetal testosterone and empathy: Evidence from the Empathy Quotient (EQ) and the 'Reading the Mind in the Eyes' Test." Social Neuroscience.
36 R846: S Jeevanandam et al. (2016). "2D:4D Ratio and its Implications in Medicine." Journal of Clinical & Diagnostic Research.
37 R1044: B Fink et al. (2007). "A preliminary investigation of the associations between digit ratio and women's perception of men's dance." Personality and Individual Differences.

38 R845: B Lenz et al. (2019). "The androgen model of suicide completion." Progress in Neurobiology.
39 R881: S Rice et al. (2018). "Adolescent and young adult male mental health: Transforming system failures into proactive models of engagement." Journal of Adolescent Health.
40 R1508: C Perez (2019). Invisible Women: Exposing Data Bias in a World Designed for Men. Chatto & Windus.
41 R743: S Bennett et al. (2023). "Male suicide and barriers to accessing professional support: A qualitative thematic analysis." Current Psychology.
42 R163: Samaritans (2020). "Out of sight, out of mind: Why less-well off, middle-aged men don't get the support they need." samaritans.org.
43 R264: L Denneson et al. (2021). "Gender differences in recovery needs after a suicide attempt: A national qualitative study of US military veterans." Medical Care.
44 R798: B Doré et al. (2017). "Helping others regulate emotion predicts increased regulation of one's own emotions and decreased symptoms of depression." Personality and Social Psychology Bulletin.
45 R699: C Emslie et al. (2006). "Men's accounts of depression: Reconstructing or resisting hegemonic masculinity?" Social Science & Medicine.
46 R1518: Merriam-Webster Dictionary (Accessed 2025). "Hegemony: Definition." merriam-webster.com.
47 R1519: R W Connell et al. (2005). "Hegemonic masculinity: Rethinking the concept." Gender & Society.
48 R699: C Emslie et al. (2006). "Men's accounts of depression: reconstructing or resisting hegemonic masculinity?" Social Science & Medicine.
49 R1029: S Tyler et al. (2022). "Suicidal ideation in the Australian construction industry: Prevalence and the associations of psychosocial job adversity and adherence to traditional masculine norms." International Journal of Environmental Research and Public Health (IJERPH).
50 R1415: The Centre for Social Justice (2025). "Lost Boys." centreforsocialjustice.org.uk.
51 R158: Samaritans (2012). "Men, suicide and society: Why disadvantaged men in midlife die by suicide." samaritans.org.
52 R647: F de Waal (2023). Different: What Apes Can Teach Us About Gender. Granta.
53 R1470: K McAuliffe (2013). "The story of the NUTS! reply." Army.mil
54 R1557: School History (Accessed 2025). "The Home Front during WWI: 1914-1918 Facts & Worksheets." schoolhistory.co.uk.
55 R1471: M Armstrong (2017). "Could the Charge of the Light Brigade have worked?" The Conversation.
56 R551: Priory (2023). "Men's mental health: 40% of men won't talk about their mental health." priorygroup.com.

PART 7
IT'S ABOUT BALANCE

Parts 2–6 have walked you through what I refer to as the 5 Dimensions of male mental health. These are all different aspects of life that I have found can help men not only to overcome crises in their life, but also to build a balanced and rewarding life. I also find that these Dimensions can offer an explanation as to why the current generic approach to mental health might not always work as well for men.

When I look at these 5 Dimensions in The ALPHA Framework, I have both a sad thought and a happy thought. My sad thought is for Brad, because he did all the things we tell men in crisis to do: he reached out for help, he went to see his doctor, he attended talking therapy, he took antidepressants, and he called his mum every evening and told her how he was feeling. But nobody Brad spoke to realised that he was spending all of his time and effort in just 1 Dimension: Achieving Recognition (which he was great at, by the way).

He wasn't Looking After Body & Mind. His testosterone was probably low (we'll never know; but he was definitely depressed). He wasn't Protecting the Cave. He had the house, he had the watch, and he had the car; but what Brad didn't have was money at the end of the month to pay for it all. He wasn't Having Adventures. Yes, he had hobbies and things he liked to do to stay motivated, but he rarely took any time off to pursue those things. Instead, he often found himself falling into bad habits. He regularly told his friends that it felt as if "*life was flying by*". And he wasn't Able to Serve. He had values and causes that he believed in, but he didn't set the time aside to support those causes in a way that made him feel useful. He regularly told his mum, Jenny, that he didn't know what the point of his life was.

Although it is too late for Brad, it is not too late for the men and boys in your life. And it is not too late for the man you are worried about. On the positive side, every man I've ever worked with is often strong when it comes to 1, 2, or 3 of these Dimensions. And if he takes the same thoughtfulness, care, and skill and applies it to the other Dimensions he might currently be neglecting, it can have a transformative effect on his mental health and on his life in general.

One of the benefits of dividing areas of life into these different Dimensions is that it gives men the opportunity to say "*Actually, I am good at that one.*" Sometimes that will be the first time they've said anything positive about themselves in quite a while. This helps them to understand what is working for them and apply it in different areas of their life.

The ALPHA Framework is not just a list of things to think about. It's not even just a list of things to talk about. It is a list of things to *do*. Because it's often the things men do that have the greatest impact on their mental health.

Ultimately, my vision is that one day in the future, when a man like Brad reaches out for help, everyone he talks to – from his doctor to his therapist to his mum – will know enough about male mental health to not simply say "*You just need to talk*". We need everyone to know that talking is vital for men, just as it is for everybody, but it is not **the solution**. It is the first step on the road to **finding the solution**. But next, men need to know what to talk about and, most importantly of all, what changes to make to take control of their life.

And if you want to know how we take all the concepts from this book and turn them into a single strategy for having supportive conversations with men and boys, that's what the final part of this book is all about.

PART 8

HOW TO TALK TO HIM

"We must stop seeing masculinity as a problem to be solved and start seeing it as a strength to be nurtured."

– Andy Cook

Supporting connection

In early 2023, after years of regularly working with, managing, and supporting men, I started attending more generic mental health training. The majority of the training focussed on listening to others, validating how they feel, and then signposting them to further support, if they needed it. It's a 3-step strategy that often goes something like:

1. Ask – Questions like "How are you feeling?" "Is everything OK?"
2. Listen – Let them share how they feel
3. Validate – Say something like "I can see why you feel that way, it must be so frustrating."

This is a fantastically simple method of supporting those who need to feel heard and who need to feel connected to someone else. The example conversation below is me using this 3-step strategy to support my wife, Emma, after a bad day at work.

> ### Example Conversation: Ryan Supporting Emma
>
> Ryan: How was your day? Are you OK?
>
> Emma: No, I'm not OK. I feel like since I started my new job, people are always telling me how I should do things. It's so frustrating.
>
> Ryan: [Says nothing but nods to show he's listening.]
>
> Emma: I know they're only trying to help, but it feels like they think that I don't know what I am doing!
>
> Ryan: I can see why you feel that way. It must be so frustrating.
>
> Emma: It really is. Thank you. I feel better just talking about it.

We haven't solved Emma's problem, but she feels better just by talking about it. Not only can this be extremely helpful, it is also very simple. I can see why this strategy is so widely taught and used!

But what would happen if I was to change my approach? This time, rather than listening to Emma, I am going to try to fix Emma's problem for her.

> ### Example Conversation: Ryan Not Supporting Emma
>
> Ryan: How was your day? Are you OK?
>
> Emma: No, I'm not OK. I feel like since I started my new job, people are always telling me how I should do things. It's so frustrating.
>
> Ryan: Next time they do that, you should say to them, "I do actually know what I am doing, thank you."
>
> Emma: I can't just say that.
>
> Ryan: Honestly, I would tell them that. Have you tried? I bet it would change things.
>
> Emma: You're not listening to me.

There was a time when this would be confusing to me. After all, if I hadn't been listening, how could I have come up with such *great* suggestions?!

But Emma doesn't feel listened to, because when she feels listened to, she feels connection, which reduces her stress – probably by causing the release of oxytocin.

While this approach may work well in many situations, there is an additional tool that I believe is vital in supporting men. Let's explore that next.

Supporting capability

I'm going to propose that we might need to tailor our approach when we are supporting men and boys, to make it more relevant to them. If I had to boil my knowledge and my experience down to a single (dramatically!) oversimplified sentence, it would be:

> ***While positive female mental health***
> ***is about feeling connected;***
> ***Positive male mental health is***
> ***about feeling capable.***

Even if I ignored everything I had learned from coaching, ignored the lived experience of hundreds of men I have worked with, and ignored all my own lived experiences as a man, we would be still be left with evidence that:

1. Oxytocin is a hormone that is released when we feel connected.
2. While oxytocin reliably reduces stress in women, it doesn't seem to consistently reduce stress in men.
3. Testosterone and serotonin reliably reduce stress in men.
4. In men, serotonin levels are associated with status and feeling successful.
5. In men, testosterone levels are associated with believing they are a winner.

I am not suggesting that women don't need to feel capable, or that men don't need to feel connected. I am simply saying that the skew is slightly different.

To me, this means that – in order to support men – we also need a simple strategy that helps men to feel capable.

And here is my 3-step strategy for doing this:

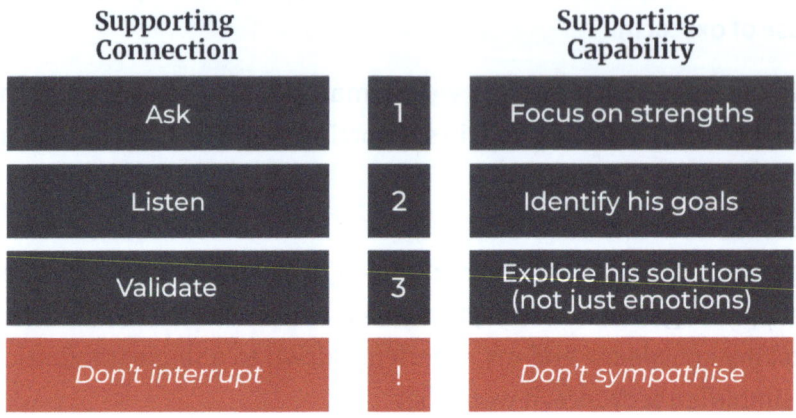

I want to show you how this works in real conversations. Some were conversations that I was a part of and some were conversations that women have told me they had with men after attending one of my workshops. We all put our own spin on the conversations. We probably stumbled over our words and were unsure what to say at times. But we followed this strategy and – most importantly – were able to support a man in his time of need.

Let's look at this strategy in action.

During a personal crisis

One Friday afternoon in 2023, I was recording a talk for an upcoming event, when my phone rang. It was a lady called Andrea who was extremely worried about her husband. Together, they had contacted all the forms of support they could think of. Andrea had called her husband's doctor, several mental health services, and listening lines (like Samaritans). Not only did the support not seem to work for her husband, but he seemed to be becoming more stressed with every phone call.

Unsure what else to do, Andrea asked her HR team at work to forward her my number (I had delivered a talk to her company a few months before). Andrea put her phone on loudspeaker so that the 3 of us could have a conversation. After the conversation, I realised I had accidentally recorded it. Andrea and her husband asked me to use the conversation in case it would help others.

Her husband is Steve, the man we met in Part 3: Looking After Body and Mind. This was our very first conversation.

Supporting Steve: How it Started...

Steve: I don't want to talk about it. I'm totally useless at everything. I know my family would be better off without me.

Ryan: I sometimes find that when men feel useless, they are having thoughts about suicide. Are you having thoughts about suicide, Steve?

[If you would like the confidence to ask that question when it matters, I would recommend you attend suicide intervention training. There are links to very economical (and some fully funded) training provided by some amazing charities available at TheMensCoach.co.uk/resources]

Steve: Yes, mate. The only reason I haven't done it is I'd probably mess that up too.

Ryan: Do you have a plan to end your life, Steve?

Steve: No, mate. I just don't want to be here.

Andrea: I'm sure you're not the only one, Steve. I'm sure there are plenty of other men who feel this way too.

Steve: Yeah. Plenty of other losers.

Why did Steve respond this way?

Andrea did what came naturally to her: she listened and tried to validate Steve's feelings. However, Steve interpreted this as sympathy, which made him feel even less capable. At this point, I decided it was important to steer the conversation in a safer direction.

> ### Supporting Steve: Focus on strengths
>
> Ryan: Can I just say, I'm really impressed with how strong you are, Steve. It takes guts to admit you're having thoughts about suicide.
>
> Steve: Thanks, mate. I didn't think of it like that.
>
> Ryan: You should. But I disagree with you – I don't think you'd mess it up. You're very capable, so I'm pleased we're talking.
>
> Steve: Thanks, mate.

What I did here was emphasise Steve's capability. I even explicitly said "You're very capable." Now it was time to identify Steve's goals.

> ### Supporting Steve: Identifying his goals
>
> Ryan: Look, Steve, suicide is always one of your options. But are you open to talking about your other options with me?
>
> Steve: Please, mate.
>
> Ryan: Well, I want to know – if you died today, what life goals would you never be able to achieve?

Steve then spent about 5 minutes discussing his various life goals, which included watching his daughter graduate, taking care of his wife, Andrea, and helping homeless kids. (Steve had been homeless in his early 20s and believed that other homeless children deserved better.) Notice that all these goals require Steve to get through his current crisis, so we are now on the same team. With his goals identified, we could move on to exploring potential solutions.

Supporting Steve: Explore his solutions (not just emotions)

Ryan: So let's make a plan to get you where you need to be in life. It's not going to be easy, but you wouldn't want it to be easy, would you?

Steve: (Laughs) No, mate, I don't want it to be easy. That would be boring.

Ryan: So what's holding you back from achieving these big goals?

Steve: *[Shared his problems with me: he was working too many hours, drinking too much, and spending more than he earned.]*

Ryan: So what do you need to do about it?

Steve: Well... I could stop work at six p.m. today and take a look at my bank statements to see if there's anything I can cut out. And I'll try a few days without booze.

[It might seem natural to sympathise with him at this point. But I didn't want to undermine the feeling of capability that Steve was experiencing. I simply said:]

Ryan: There's the man I knew I was talking to. I know you are capable of making it happen, but who could help by providing you with support and accountability?

Andrea: I wish you could see Steve now, Ryan. All the colour has come back to his face. I've got my husband back.

This transcript has been shortened and simplified, but the entire conversation with Steve lasted less than 11 minutes. Probably 6 minutes of it was Steve telling me about his life goals. By the end of the call, Steve was so excited that he had to leave to start working on his goals. Before he left, we made a plan as to what Steve can do if he feels this way again.

I wanted to start with this example so that we can directly address what you might feel is the biggest risk: that the man you are worried about might be thinking about taking his own life.

I also want you to know that if you are worried a conversation about suicide might give someone the idea of taking their own life, the evidence says the opposite. It's been found that conversations about suicide are actually protective. And younger people tend to benefit more from exposure to conversations about suicide.[1]

And if Steve had reacted with "No, mate. I'm not thinking about that", there would have been no harm done. It would also have been a relief to Andrea!

I don't want to use the cliché here that you "*can't make it worse*," because that is always a possibility. I'll say again that you can get relevant training if it's likely you will come into contact with someone who might be having thoughts about suicide. Such training shows you how to bring up difficult conversations and focus on the person's needs. The purpose of this section of the book is not to train you to have conversations about suicide, but to complement the training that is available while adding a new tool to your existing communication skills and instincts.

Four weeks later, Steve and I were on Zoom call together for his first coaching call, and his focus shifted to his physical health (as we explored in Part 3: Looking After Body & Mind).

Dealing with disappointment

Debbie was working away from home when she received a text from her 17-year-old son, David. It was not good news. Despite his best efforts, David had just heard that his dream university had rejected his application. She parked her car next to the hotel she would be staying in and called David as quickly as she could. Here is the overall gist of their conversation.

Supporting David

Debbie: I've been really impressed with how well you handled things since you got the news from the uni. I think they're going to regret their decision because you're going to achieve a lot in the future!

David: Thanks. I just did what I had to do after I found out what was happening.

> Debbie: I'm sure there are lots of other universities who are looking for someone like you, so what are you thinking of doing next?
>
> David: I don't know really. I had my heart set on that place so I don't really have a Plan B.
>
> Debbie: You might not need this but if you're free tomorrow night, we could have a chat and look at the different options together, then make a plan.
>
> David: Thanks, that would be helpful.

Once Debbie was back from her work trip, she and David spent an evening talking through the other university options. Another university did accept him, he just had to make a few more applications. And even if there had been no other university to accept him, he would have found another path forwards, I am sure.

The reason I know how the conversation went is because Debbie told me. A few weeks before she had to support David after he got the news from university, she'd attended one of my workshops where she learned this 3-step strategy. She stayed behind to talk to me, and promised to let me know how she got on. At first, she was reluctant to have a conversation with David that wasn't about emotions.

After this conversation, however, she was confident that it was a useful tool for her. While she was debriefing me on what happened, she told me how these conversations normally went.

Using 'Ask, Listen, Validate' on David

> Debbie: I'm worried about you. Are you OK?
>
> David: Yes. It kind of sucks, but I'm fine.
>
> Debbie: How do you feel about it?

> David: Yeah, well it sucks but it's one of those things. We have to get on with life.
>
> Debbie: It must be so hard for you, David.
>
> David: No, it's fine. I'm fine.

Normally, David shuts down the conversation. I believe that men and boys have become well-practised at shutting down conversations which are well-intentioned, but don't help them to feel more capable. They might even be trying to prevent an increase in oxytocin, which could make them feel more stressed (as we saw in the 'hug study' - see Part 4: Protecting the Cave).

Talking about dangerous driving

This is an example of a conversation with a young man who is driving everywhere so fast he is in danger of causing a serious accident.

> **Talking About Dangerous Behaviour**
>
> You have great control of your car, but not all other drivers do.
>
> If you were driving quickly and someone pulled out in front of you, you could lose your car, your driver's licence, and your job.
>
> I know it takes discipline but would you be willing to stick to the speed limit to keep those freedoms?

I know that this conversation worked because I was the young man on the receiving end of these words. At the time I was 22 years old, I drove everywhere like I was on a racetrack, and it was a miracle I hadn't had a bad accident – although I had come close many times.

I had been approached before by people who wanted me to take more care when driving. But when they started by telling me how worried they were, what I heard was "*You're not capable of controlling a fast car*". And I would prove that I was… by driving faster.

Then, I was approached by my manager at work who used these words. Because he started by addressing that I had some skills when it came to car control, I felt no need to shut down or blow up like I had when others tried to have this conversation with me. He presumed that my goals were keeping my car, my licence, and my job. He was correct. And the solution he offered was to slow down to lower the risk of losing them by having a bad accident.

By that point, this manager had been working with young men, who all had nice company cars, for about 10 years. I wonder how many times he had used those exact words… They worked, and I made a conscious effort to drive slower.

Encouraging boys (and men) to help with tasks

If I was going to use this 3-step strategy to ask for help from a man, I would probably use phrases like these.

Encouraging Boys (and Men) to Help with Tasks

[Focus on strengths] I need someone strong enough to carry furniture and skilled with a drill.

[Identify his goals] I know you like to practise your skills, so…

[Explore his solutions] When we move house next month, can we count on you to help?

Each one is short, straight to the point, and will make him feel useful and capable.

And here's an example of my wife, Emma, getting me to help with a household task.

We had a pumpkin on the kitchen counter that needed to be cut up. I had planned to do it but had never gotten around to it. Emma would routinely remind me, saying "*That pumpkin I asked you to cut up is still on the side.*"

> ### Emma Asking Ryan to Perform a Task
>
> Emma: That pumpkin I asked you to cut up is still on the side. Do you know when you'll be able to cut it up?
>
> Ryan: Yeah, I know. I'll cut it up when I get a chance.

This went on for about 2 weeks. Then one day as we arrived back from a walk in the woods, Emma changed her strategy.

> ### Making Ryan Feel Incapable
>
> Emma: I'm going to ask your friend Lee if he'll cut up that pumpkin on the side for the dog.
>
> Ryan: What? Why would you ask Lee? I'm perfectly capable of cutting up a pumpkin. Where is it?
>
> [30 seconds later, the pumpkin was cut into pieces.]

The reason I'm sharing this is that, while it's a bit jovial and light-hearted, there's a serious message here. Emma knew exactly what she was doing, because she knows me so well.

I believe that every time we make a man feel incapable, we're going to get a reaction. That reaction could range from him shutting down the conversation, driving fast to prove he can, or deciding not to reach out for help again. But there is going to be a reaction. In this instance, it was simply some (long overdue) pumpkin cutting.

When to support connection and when to support capability

If you're ever unsure which approach to use, the best person to ask is the one you're supporting! Just ask directly with a sincere tone:

"I want to support in the way that is most useful to you. If you'd like to get it off your chest, I'm here to listen. If you'd like to find a solution, I can ask some practical questions. Which would be best for this situation?"

This question appreciates that different people benefit from different support at different times. Notice that neither approach involves giving advice – they are both about listening and supporting, but in subtly different ways.

One challenge men often face when reaching out for help is that there's only one option, and it's probably not the one they are looking for.

More supportive statements and questions

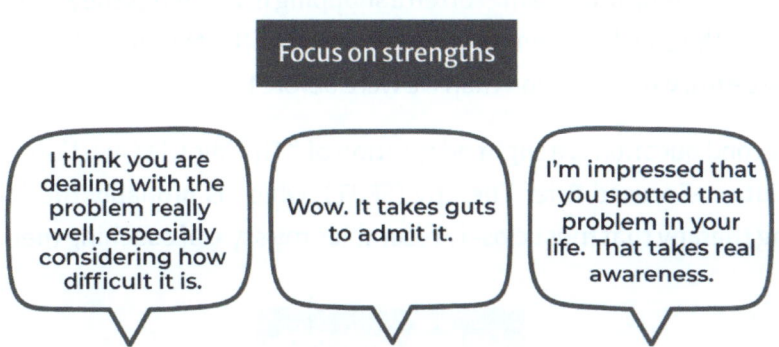

It can be a knee-jerk reaction to say something like "I'm so sorry to hear that" when someone tells us that they are stressed or have an issue in their life. For men, I would recommend instead focussing on the fact that they told you in itself being a strength that they have. None of these statements even require you to know the man you are supporting, they are simply focussing on talking as being a sign of strength.

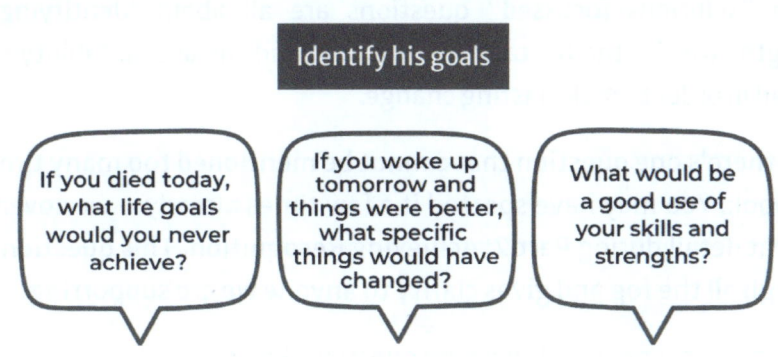

You'll recognise the first question as the one I asked Steve, but I use it a lot. Because of the way that this question is phrased, almost any answer gives us something we can work with. It's not only useful when men are having thoughts about suicide; you can use it as a way to quickly and efficiently identify life goals wherever that would be beneficial. I am often asked in workshops "What happens if they say 'Nothing, I have nothing I want to achieve'?"

Firstly, it hasn't happened yet. Everyone I have ever asked this question to has shared something important – often a shopping list of things they need to do! But when the day does come and a man replies with "Nothing", I don't think we will be in a worse position than we were before I asked.

The second question is a slight adaptation of "The Miracle Question" – part of Solution-Focused Brief Therapy (SFBT), which is probably the form of talking therapy that most closely resembles my style of coaching men.

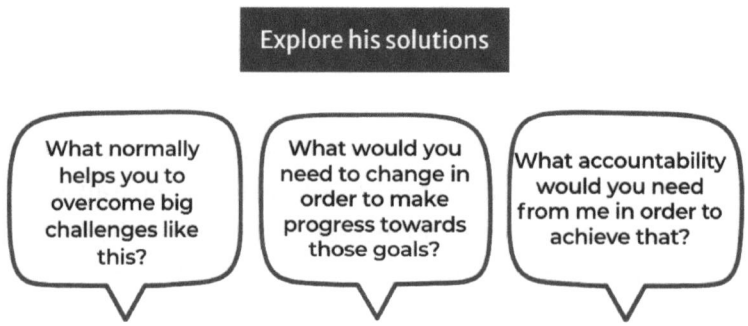

These "solutions-focussed" questions are all about identifying the strengths within, the obstacles in the way, and the accountability that's needed in order to make lasting change.

Then there's one question that cannot be mentioned too many times in this book. You may have spotted it a few times already – we covered it in great detail during Part 2: Achieving Recognition. This question cuts through all the fog and gives clarity to anyone we are supporting.

This is the most powerful coaching question I know.

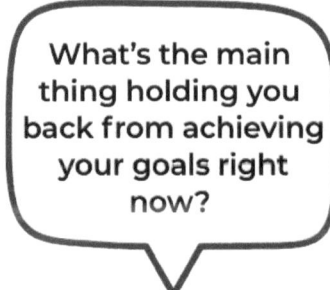

Recommended word swaps

If your objective is to engage men (or boys), it's important to use the words they use. This is common practice in marketing, business, making friends – almost every arena of life. But sometimes, when it comes to mental health and wellbeing, men are expected to use words they often don't identify with.

I'm very aware that words are subjective, and most of my work is with UK men who speak English as their first language, but even so, here are some word swaps that I have found work very well when it comes to engaging men.

Rather than	Try instead
How do you feel?	What's on your mind?
Open up	Team up
Talk about how you feel	Talk about solutions
Struggling	Stressed
Self-love / Self-care	Self-maintenance
Male-dominated	Majority-male
Vulnerable	Authentic
I love you	I am impressed by you

"How do you feel?" → "What's on your mind?"

These might appear to be the same question, but I find "What's on your mind?" elicits a more detailed response, giving him (and you) more to work with. Ironically, the answer to "What's on your mind?" almost always includes how they feel anyway, plus a whole lot more.

"Open up" → "Team up"

Many men now feel under societal pressure to "open up" which they might not associate with being helpful. I suggest replacing this with "team up" has the same focus on support but from a more positive and collaborative perspective.

"Talk about how you feel" → "Talk about solutions"

Talking is vital for men, but it's vital we don't see it as "the solution". Instead, it is the first step on the road to finding their solution. So why not appreciate that and invite them to "talk about solutions"? It's a practical offer that I find men are often keen to take up. This also combines fittingly with the previous word swap. Rather than "I think it would really benefit you to open up and talk about how you feel", try "How about we team up and talk about solutions?"

"Struggling" → "Stressed"

When talking about men we are worried about, there is a tendency to use words like "struggling". I believe this is quite stigmatising as it suggests that the person in question is not capable. Conversely, although the word "stressed" has a similar meaning, men are able to identify when they are stressed and may be motivated to engage with support that offers to resolve stress. [2]

"Self-love" / "Self-care" → Self-maintenance

While these concepts can overlap, the "self-love / self-care" concept can be seen as "woolly" for some men. "Self-maintenance", on the other hand, is a clear term that prompts conversations about the necessity of sleep, healthy food, rest, time off, paying off debt – all the positive and productive things we often need men to do to support their wellbeing.

"Male-dominated" → "Majority-male"

There are some instances where the term "male-dominated" is completely appropriate. But it is often misused to simply refer to an industry, organisation, or group that are mainly male. In this case, I find the term "majority-male" avoids the connotations of domination, and the idea that one sex must dominate the other. Likewise, "majority-female" is, I think, often much more appropriate than "female-dominated".

"Vulnerable" → "Authentic"

There is a lot of societal pressure on men today to be "vulnerable". It's important to know that when many men hear the term vulnerable, they associate it with its literal meaning – Merriam-Webster defines vulnerable as "*capable of being physically or emotionally wounded; open to attack or damage*". When you look at its literal meaning, I don't think we actually want anyone to be vulnerable, including the men we care about. I am a big fan of Brené Brown and her pioneering work, but often when you hear Brené talking about being *vulnerable*, you could argue that she is really talking about being "*authentic*". Merriam-Webster defines authentic as "*not false or imitation; true to one's own personality, spirit, or character; worthy of acceptance or belief as conforming to or based on fact*". It seems to me that this is what many people now mean when they use the word "vulnerable". And the good news is that men understand this concept more accurately.

"I love you" → "I am impressed by you"

This one is a little light-hearted, but a few years ago I mentioned to my wife, Emma, that when she says something I have done is impressive, I get a warm feeling inside, and feel like I belong. "That's how I feel when you say 'I love you'!" Emma replied. A few weeks later, I told this story to the chief executive of an international company. When I next met her, she told me that meetings with her male subordinates had totally transformed since she tried starting them by picking something impressive they had done lately. She said that they had become a lot more open and collaborative, with just that one genuine comment.

How to help him to find the right support

It's also very possible that – as much as you care – you might not be the best person to support him. And that's OK too.

There have been many moments in my life where I have realised that I can't support my closest friends or family the way that I can support my coaching clients. I'm just too close and too emotionally involved to offer the non-judgemental space that they need.

It's not that men don't talk, it's just that certain conditions need to be in place first. In my experience, men naturally team up with others when they:

1. **Trust** they won't be made to feel less capable,
2. **Respect** the other person's ability to help, and
3. **Know** they won't be a burden to others.

For example, when I work with organisations that have driving instructors (emergency service providers or logistics companies, for instance), the instructors often become confidants for the men they are training. But not on the first day; this usually happens after a few days, when the men are starting to master a new skill.

The conditions are perfect. The learner **trusts** his instructor, having already experienced the psychological safety of the learning environment. He **respects** his instructor's ability to help, because that has already been demonstrated. And he **knows** he won't be a burden, as they are stuck in a vehicle together with a job to do! Add to that, they are sitting side by side, without intense eye contact, making the exchange of information far more likely.

So while the HR team are claiming that "men don't talk" because the "Time to Talk" coffee morning was empty again, the driving instructors are being used as talking therapists (whether they like it or not) every day of the week!

In coaching I create these conditions by talking through The ALPHA Framework for over an hour with clients before we begin The Future Call. This means we have discussed issues like suicide, success, testosterone, security, addictions and purpose. We've discussed the various signs of stress and science-based strategies. By the point the Future Call begins, the trust, respect and knowledge is in place. What follows is courage, honesty and authenticity.

The best thing you can do is to ask him *"What kind of support would work best for you?"* This could be in a therapy session, coaching session, or simply a long drive with a friend, colleague, or partner. Men's support groups can be excellent for some men, as they can provide this kind of environment. But I would always start by asking him what he needs, and what he thinks will work best for him.

ENDNOTES

1. R924: T Dazzi et al. (2014). "Does asking about suicide and related behaviours induce suicidal ideation? What is the evidence?" Psychological Medicine.
2. R1011: C Stein (2018). "Mind Your Language: How Men Talk About Mental Health." Men's Health Forum.

FINAL THOUGHTS

It is June 2025, 6 years after I first heard the news about Brad.

I've just returned from a walk through the woods next to my apartment. On my way back I took a detour to walk past the bench that now displays Brad's name on a commemorative plaque. As I emerged from the woods, I walked under the hornbeam trees where I saw Jenny 6 years ago. I can still see the tears that streamed down her cheeks as she told me the news about Brad. But Jenny doesn't live here any more. She couldn't bear to live in the same house in which she'd brought up her son.

It hit me today what an unplanned but amazing journey I've been on since I heard the news about Brad. I'm struck by how many other men I've met during that time who were in a similar situation to Brad, and women in a similar situation to Jenny. I hope that I've been able to offer them some useful tools and insights.

As I said at the very start of this book, The ALPHA Framework started off as a plan for myself, fulfilling a promise I made to Jenny to learn more about male mental health. The very start of that research took me somewhere I hadn't even anticipated, reframing my entire understanding of male mental health and wellbeing. I wanted to put all that research into a practical model I could use to keep me accountable. I didn't think it would be relevant to anyone else. Seeing the difference it was making in my own life was enough for other men around me to start asking me whether they could use it too. Then women wanted to know how they could use this Framework to support the men in their lives.

By this point I was only working with individuals, but the men I was working with started recommending me to their colleagues and therapists, and before I knew it, I was invited to speak about The ALPHA Framework on stage. That's when I started to believe that maybe this Framework was relevant across the UK. Then I started being invited to other countries to explain the Framework around the world.

What's most interesting of all here is how The ALPHA Framework isn't something I learned from university or from a mental health course I went on. As I said to Christopher when we first met, it's been created from scientific articles that are available to anyone with a library card. It's been honed from the conversations with men who probably would have spoken to anyone who took a genuine interest and wanted to discuss practical solutions, rather than focussing solely on emotions.

And if I can do all this without going to university, with nothing more than a library card, a Zoom licence, and some open-minded curiosity, imagine what the healthcare systems, mental health services, and policy makers could do with this information.

And more importantly, imagine what you can do with it.

I'm excited about the difference you can make to the man you're worried about, now you know how to help him…

NEXT STEPS

Thank you page

Thank you to the women in my life who made this book and my work possible.

Thank you to my mum, Louise, for raising me to be curious about the world.

Thank you, Emma Weaver, for your constant guidance and encouragement.

Thank you, Debbie Roberts, for convincing me that my experience and knowledge could be useful to others.

Thank you, Debbie Jenkins, for the moment of clarity that led to this book.

Most importantly, thank you to my beautiful wife, Emma, for believing in me, then giving me the opportunity and accountability to pursue my purpose in life.

There is no greater gift.

How to test Testosterone Levels

Because many men are interested in testosterone—and because improving testosterone naturally involves improving metabolic health—I believe that better education around testosterone would reduce the number of men dying from preventable issues.

Here are some things you might want to know about testing testosterone in men:

1. How to test

Testing is straightforward. In most countries you can order a home finger-prick test or visit a clinic to have blood taken.

2. When to test

The best time is within a few hours of waking, before eating, as that's when testosterone is naturally highest. Clinics often recommend 9 a.m., but that assumes he sleeps at night and wakes in the morning. For men working night shifts, 9 a.m. would be the wrong time. What matters most is consistency: testing at the same time of day so results can give a good comparison.

3. Which markers to test

If the test is arranged by a healthcare professional, they will be able to advise which markers are most relevant. In my coaching programmes, I use tests that include:

- Total Testosterone (serum testosterone): the overall amount of testosterone in the blood. This is the measure I usually refer to throughout this book.
- Luteinising Hormone (LH): the brain's signal to the testes to produce testosterone. This helps show whether low testosterone is due to a problem with the brain's signalling or with the testes themselves.
- Free Testosterone: the small fraction not bound to proteins such as SHBG or albumin. This is the active portion doing testosterone's work in the body.

Some professionals suggest that free testosterone is most important, but in my experience, total testosterone is the most useful marker for men's metabolic health. Still, all of these markers have value, and it's important not to oversimplify them.

All of these markers (total testosterone, LH and free testosterone) can be significantly increased with the lifestyle changes in Part 3: Looking After Body & Mind.

4. How often to test

Testosterone can fluctuate quickly (think of football fans during the 1994 World Cup), so one result is only a snapshot. But several results over time can reveal important trends. When I make lifestyle changes, I test every three months. Otherwise, one or two tests a year are enough to keep me accountable and looking after myself.

5. Which test to buy

On my website (TheMensCoach.co.uk/resources) I share the test I believe offers the best value for UK men. I base this on cost, the markers included, and ease of use. I don't take commission for these recommendations, because I want testing to be as affordable and accessible as possible.

6. The problem with just testing

While testosterone testing can be a useful tool, it can also create problems if it isn't combined with good education around testosterone. Because the reference range for testosterone is now so low, many men are told their levels are "normal" when in reality they are very low compared to what was typical just a few decades ago. This can make men complacent about their health when actually they would benefit from the right changes.

On the other hand, some men are told they have low testosterone but aren't made aware of how much testosterone can often be improved through lifestyle changes. That can leave them believing testosterone replacement therapy (TRT) is their only answer. And while TRT can address the symptoms of low testosterone, it isn't directly addressing the cause.

But when testosterone testing is paired with education, it becomes an easy and economical way for men to track their wellbeing and take charge of positive changes.

ABOUT RYAN PARKE

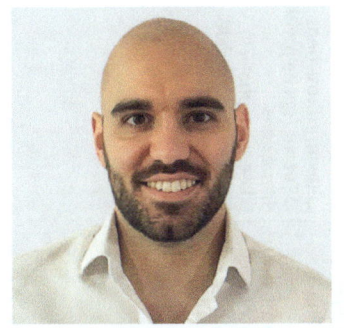

Ryan Parke is The Men's Coach – a TEDx Speaker specialising in how hormones, lifestyle, and goal setting impact male mental health. Having created an evidence-based framework drawing on over 1,000 sources and his extensive coaching experience, Ryan works with industry leaders, international schools, emergency service providers, and NHS Trusts who want to make support more inclusive, engaging, and effective for men.

Alongside his real-world coaching experience, Ryan is also an international award-winning speaker and a Professional Member of the Professional Speaking Association. He is a trained Mental Health First Aider, Suicide First Aider, and Men's Health Champion, with Samaritans training in suicide prevention.

The ALPHA Framework
Quick Reference Guide

	A Achieving Recognition	**L** Looking After Body & Mind	**P** Protecting the Cave	**H** Having Adventures	**A** Able to Serve
	Serotonin	Testosterone	Security	Dopamine	Purpose
Signs of Stress	- Feeling *stuck or unsuccessful* - Lack of written goals - Outcome-based goals - Comparison with others - Loss of social status (redundancy, retirement)	- Feeling *down, depressed* - Low energy, poor sleep - Poor prostate health - High blood pressure - Poor heart health - Type 2 diabetes - Low libido, ED	- Feeling *overwhelmed* - Feeling *hopeless or ashamed* - Financial uncertainty - Relationship insecurity - Feeling *like a burden*	- Life flying by - Lack of motivation - Working all the time - Procrastination - Distractions / cravings (e.g. porn, alcohol, social media, etc.)	- Feeling *useless* - Feeling *unfulfilled* - Wondering *what is the point of life?* - Loss of child contact - Death feels meaningful or heroic
Science-based Strategies	☐ Write down life goals ☐ Identify obstacles ☐ Set weekly goals ☐ Weekly goals should be small, effort-based and wholly within your control ☐ Arrange weekly accountability	☐ Real food: reduce carbs, increase natural fats ☐ Sleep: 7–8 hours/day ☐ Exercise: 150+ mins a week ☐ Vitamin D3 (sunlight, supplements, natural fat) ☐ Reduce / stop alcohol ☐ Watch team wins	☐ Express and address underlying issues ☐ Review monthly costs ☐ Focus on building a monthly surplus ☐ Team up with money / debt charities (if needed) ☐ Spend quality time with partner (if relevant)	☐ Take time to 'recharge' ☐ Explore new places and skills ☐ Identify distractions ☐ Cut out / get help with distractions ☐ Use smartphone in black and white mode	☐ Identify skills and strengths ☐ Serve people / causes that matter most ☐ Support family, friends and faith ☐ Be part of a team ☐ Say 'no' to unfulfilling things

TheMensCoach.co.uk | The ALPHA Framework™ | © YKIWYSI Limited 2025 | Version 5.0 UK Edition

MENTAL HEALTH SUPPORT

In an emergency, call one of these numbers

For urgent mental health support, stop reading this book and reach out to one of the organisations below:

If you're based in the UK, call 999 in life-threatening emergencies, including if someone is attempting suicide. If the situation is not life-threatening, dial 111 and select option 2 for mental health support.

If it would help to feel listened to, you can call the **Samaritans** confidentially and free of charge any time on 116 123.

Befrienders Worldwide – Provide international support for those having thoughts about suicide. Help is available in 193 countries and 44 different languages. Visit **befrienders.org** and select your country from the home page.

Papyrus – Offers free non-judgemental UK phone, text, and web-chat support for young people having thoughts about suicide, and those worried about young people. Visit **papyrus-uk.org**

The Hub of Hope – The UK's largest mental health support database, providing you with local mental health, NHS, youth, and peer support based on your postcode. Visit **hubofhope.co.uk**

RYAN'S RESOURCES PAGE

Ryan's Resources page provides contact details for organisations that provide:

- Urgent mental health support
- Local UK specialist support
- Support with money & debt problems
- Tips for managing your mobile
- Suicide intervention training
- Useful home blood tests
- Information on diet and nutrition
- Information on female health and hormones
- Useful tools for healthcare practitioners
- Help with testosterone levels
- Engaging speakers on the subjects of mental health, wellbeing, and inclusion

Visit TheMensCoach.co.uk/resources